About The Author

Joan Crank was born and raised in South Liverpool before moving to Billinge, St.Helens in 1965. A wife and mother of two daughters, As a mature student, Joan qualified to be a Nursery Nurse. She worked on the Children's Ward at Billinge Hospital for over 20 years before retirement.

Joan cared for her husband Dave for over 10 years. He was diagnosed with Alzheimer's in 2002 and sadly passed away in 2012.

Throughout her life, Joan has always been very pro-active in fund raising for her local community and is highly regarded for her humour, warmth and vitality.

Always Look On The Bright Side…

Our Travels with Alzheimer's

By Joan Crank

Published by St Helens Carers Centre

First Published in Great Britain in 2014 by
St Helens Carers Centre

ISBN 978-0-9928138-0-2

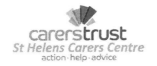

carerstrust
St Helens Carers Centre
action · help · advice

St Helens Carers Centre
31-35 Baldwin Street
St Helens
WA10 2RS

www.StHelensCarers.org.uk

Acknowledgements

This book would not have been possible without the guidance, help and support of the editor, and my friend, Sue Pierlewski. Thank you so much Sue for your patience while also caring for Rhys (also living with Alzheimer's disease). You are amazing.

Thanks to my daughter Sue, son-in-law Wayne and grandchildren Matt, Sophie and Jess. Also my other daughter Jane, son-in-law Paul and grandchildren Millie and Annie, not forgetting Pippin the dog. Even from a distance you have given me so much love and support both during your Dad's illness and since he passed away.

To the lovely Fairclough family, thanks for all those Sunday dinners followed by fun and laughter which Dave loved. Special thanks to Alex Fairclough Bell for reading drafts of the book as it went along and sending me encouraging e-mails.

Thanks so much to Derek and Ella, Barbara and Paul and all the Crank family for your regular visits which often turned into sing-alongs. Your support has been and, still is wonderful.

To all my friends and neighbours in Billinge for continuing to include Dave and I in all social occasions even when we struggled, and for taking Dave on walks, giving me a break.

Doctor Frances, Dave's consultant, for all those years of caring and also the staff at the Memory Clinic, thank you so much.

Jeanette, Dave's Community Psychiatric Nurse. You were more than a nurse, you became like a friend and your visits were down on the calendar and regarded as an activity for the afternoon.

To Aaron, a great carer, and also to Doreen and Marie from Crossroads Card. Thanks for all the fun and laughter.

Joanne Hornby Carer Support Officer at St Helens Carers Centre for your support and help over the years.

Kim from 'Age U.K'. Thanks for arranging the art lessons with Bill (so sorry Dave ran off Bill but you did try hard).

Carol and Joan (trustees of the Hargreaves Dementia Trust) for your help and support.

Finally I am so grateful to Alan Ashton, Chief Executive of St. Helens Carers Centre and his team for all their hard work, expertise and enthusiasm in helping publishing this book. They certainly went that extra mile.

The profits from the sale of this book will be donated to the local charities that supported both Joan and Dave; St Helens MIND, St Helens Alzheimer's Activity Group and St Helens Carers Centre.

Contents

Chapter 1

GETTING A DIAGNOSIS

Dave and I sat in a crowded waiting room feeling a little nervous, waiting to be called in to see a doctor who would give us the results of a brain scan which Dave had undergone a couple of weeks previously at Liverpool Royal Hospital. We had known for a couple of years that things hadn't been right. We were hoping to get an explanation for Dave's recent behaviour and mood swings, and that it would be a diagnosis which would be followed up with some kind of treatment or surgery. Dave was called in first to see the doctor. I had no idea what had been said to Dave previously but he looked extremely nervous as I was asked to sit down beside him. The doctor seemed as nervous as we were; clearly he hadn't had a lot of experience in breaking bad news to people, or at least to someone as young and healthy looking as Dave, who was sixty at the time.

'Your husband has a condition… that I cannot treat. I will refer him to a department a Consultant in old age psychiatric conditions will be able to treat him.'

'Do you know what this condition is?' I asked as Dave and I grasped each other's hands.

'Dementia,' he said, as if relieved to get the word out.

I can still hear the sharp intake of breath from Dave as I write this. I wanted to cuddle him and tell him it was a mistake and it would all be okay. I knew it wouldn't be.

The next thing, we were out of the door looking at a sea of faces in a very crowded waiting room in total shock. I can't remember seeing the nurse again. No one to ask if we would be alright. No offer of counselling when we had just been given the most devastating news of our lives, when we had recently begun to plan our retirement after a lifetime of hard work.

Sitting in the car on the hospital car park, both in tears, we tried to absorb the news. Dave asked if I would drive home, which was a relief to me as driving had become a problem.

'Hang on Dave,' I said, 'all they've done is give it a name. Let's think positively, take this one day at a time and find out about medication, diet, therapies etc.'

When we got home I rang the hospital and asked to speak to the doctor we had seen that morning.

'Are we talking about Alzheimer's disease?' I asked him.

'Yes,' he said, 'early onset.'

It took a phone call to finally know what we were dealing with. Getting this diagnosis had been like pulling teeth.

So, the battle would commence the following day. But, for now, we had to break the shattering news to our two lovely daughters and their families, Dave's family with whom he was very close, plus my own family and all of our friends.

Chapter 2

BREAKING THE NEWS

We talked things through as much as we could. We thought about telling our girls, Sue and Jane, and then of course we both dissolved into tears.

Sue and her family lived in Singapore at the time, and Sue must have felt so helpless being so far away from us. But then again it was a case of now we know what we are dealing with so let's find out about available treatment.

Jane and her family live in Hampshire but I'm sure it felt as far away as Singapore on that day. Two very sad tearful phone calls but, as far away as they both were, they couldn't have been more supportive.

The next step was to tell Dave's siblings. His elder brother, Derek, lived just a few miles away. When we arrived they were in the garden. It was such a sunny day and Derek was sweeping up leaves. His wife, Ella, offered to make a drink but I asked her to sit down while we told them both the news.

Ella's response was, 'Well, thank God it's not a brain tumour.'

Derek carried on sweeping giving no eye contact.

'What happens next?' he asked, showing no emotion but his body language said it all.

He agreed to inform Barbara, Dave's younger sister, and her husband Paul, who has since told me she was shocked as she didn't think anyone so young could develop Alzheimer's at such an early age. A misconception held by many people.

It was agreed that Dave's younger brother, Edward, could be told in a couple of weeks when he came up for Barbara and Paul's son's wedding. (When the wedding occurred, Edward was devastated when he was told and asked if money would help and if we could get the drugs more quickly by buying them privately.)

So we had had what seemed like a never ending morning and when we got home it was to a phone call from our friends Pat and Arthur, asking us to come around for a BBQ lunch. It was the last thing I felt like but as Pat said, 'You have to eat. It's just the four of us, so come round and let's sit in the garden.'

We were a little subdued at first but eventually we relaxed into a pleasant afternoon. Our friend, Marj rang and Pat passed the phone to me - another difficult phone call to a shocked friend. I asked Marj to pass the news on to our circle of friends. We had all been friends for thirty years so I knew the effect the news would have.

As we were leaving Pat hugged Dave and said, 'Until I see you up a tree in one of Joan's frocks I'm not going to worry about you.'

Dave laughed heartily. His sense of humour was to be his saving grace. The song, 'Always Look on the Bright Side of Life', was to become his theme tune.

We were exhausted but needed to wind down with what I thought should be an encouraging chat before going to bed. We talked things through truthfully… Okay, things didn't look good but nothing bad was going to happen overnight. We had already been told there were new drugs that would slow it down. 'We'll take one day at a time', I said. 'We won't sit at home and mope'.

The key words in our lives were to be ACCEPTANCE and GRATITUDE. Acceptance that after a long period of tests and examinations, a scan on the brain had revealed Alzheimer's and we would have to learn to deal with it as best we could. Gratitude that we had a loving family and friends to support us, (little did we know then how many more friends we were to make through support groups), and gratitude also for a strong faith and a sense of humour which was to be our saviour on many an occasion. So we went to bed feeling positive, or so I thought.

'Cuddle my back, Joan.' said Dave.

So we did 'spoons' and then I heard him crying softly and I joined him.

Chapter 3

THE FIRST PRESCRIPTION

I needed to find out when we would get the appointment to have Dave's drugs prescribed. I rang the number I had been given and was shocked when the phone was answered with the response, 'Department for Old Age Psychiatry'. Dave was only sixty.

I asked when we could expect Dave to be prescribed Aricept (the drug which would slow down Dave's condition.) 'He'll have to have an aptitude test first,' I was told.

'When will that be?

'Well, the nurse practitioner who does the aptitude tests is off sick,' she said.

Will she be back soon?'

'No, she's off on long term sick so we're looking around ten weeks'.

I had a feeling of panic inside. 'That's totally unacceptable'. I said.

Knowing things had been going from bad to worse for the last couple of years I wanted Dave to be on his medication straight away.

'A few more weeks isn't going to make much difference', she said. I asked if there was anyone else I could speak to and was told there wasn't until he'd had his aptitude test. I did not like her attitude and had no hesitation in deciding to write to the Community Health Council and it was to be a strong letter of complaint.

Within a week we had a letter with an appointment to see Dr Frances (who Dave came to regard as a great friend over the last ten years). She prescribed 'Aricept' and told Dave he would remain on it for life. Dr Frances was to be Dave's consultant. That day she was a beacon of hope.

Mini Mental Test

Aptitude tests became something Dave dreaded. They had to be done on a regular basis to see whether the drug was still effective and also to monitor his emotional state and the effect on me. This would stress both of us. Dave, because he thought he was being judged, would desperately try to practise answers. We would be sitting in the waiting room and he would say to me 'What's the doctor's name? What's the name of this building? What day is it, etc?'

The feeling of relief when it was over was immense. I, in turn, had feelings of anxiety and disloyalty as I filled in the form given to me regarding his behaviour at home. He was becoming increasingly aggressive and I found it hard admitting this, as I knew it wasn't Dave but was the effect and frustration of what his illness was doing to him. Even so, I knew the importance of being truthful regarding his behaviour, and yet the guilt was so hard. Something I was going to learn to live with.

Chapter 4

THE ACCIDENT

A couple of years previously, Dave had had an accident at work in which a fork lift truck had shed an unsafe load on him while he was doing a maintenance job. He was taken to hospital where it was discovered he had injuries to the cartilages in his chest and ankle. When I arrived to take him home he had an oxygen mask on. Although I believe he was knocked unconscious he was never given a brain scan. The person discharging him said he was fit to go and there was no need for a follow up appointment. That night, in bed, he was having panic attacks and hyperventilating. I can categorically say that to me Dave was never the same from that night onwards.

After six months off sick and being prescribed an anti-depressant he took early retirement when the company agreed to release his pension. They had already accepted liability and the union had provided us with a solicitor. Legal advice or not it was all too much for Dave. After months of appointments and making statements etc. an offer of £2,000 was made followed by another offer of £8,000. This was accepted, against the advice of the solicitor, but to settle out of court seemed the only way to give Dave peace of mind. In recent years I tried to re-open the case but was sent a copy of a hand written letter of Dave's acknowledging receipt of the cheque and saying that he would not be making any further claim. Ironically that would be one of the last legible letters Dave was to write as Alzheimer's was soon to claim his literacy skills.

I asked Dr. Frances if in her opinion the accident could have caused Dave's condition but she said it would be difficult to prove. Would more compensation have helped with what was happening to him? I don't think so. We would count our blessings instead of money.

Chapter 5

DRIVING

An immediate problem was the issue of Dave's ability to drive. Dr Frances arranged for him to have neurological tests and then an actual driving test. He found all this very traumatic.

When Dave returned from his driving test the examiner and colleague were chatting positively, which made Dave feel he was going to be fine. Unfortunately, when he then received his letter asking him to return his licence the reason given was, 'due to the unpredictability of his condition'. Why give him hope? Why, if the condition is so unpredictable, can some people drive and some not? Shouldn't all patients once diagnosed have their doctors inform the DVLA? I am not being flippant here but I do know how devastated he was when he lost his licence.

In fact, I suffered almost as much when he became my passenger. He turned into the worst back seat driver I've ever known, accusing me of over steering when we went around corners, constantly telling me I was going the wrong way and sometimes trying to change gear for me. However, he settled down eventually.

'What have you got to do?' I would say.

'Trust you', he would reply, or sometimes, 'I don't know; I've got Alzheimer's.'

He never lost his sense of humour and he soon accepted
that I was his chauffeur.

Chapter 6

DISCOVERING THE ALZHEIMER'S SOCIETY

One day we decided to have a day out to Southport where we could either walk the promenade or just amble around the shops [something he once hated but had now begun to like]. Dave wanted to look in the golf shop, which fortuitously happened to be opposite the local branch of the Alzheimer's Society. While he was browsing in the shop I tentatively approached the office and rang the bell. The door was opened by Annie, our first new friend in the world of support workers. I explained that Dave was in the shop opposite and that I was unsure how he would feel about me seeking help already.

So we stood in the doorway chatting casually, watching out for Dave coming out of the golf shop. She told me when and where the next Alzheimer's meeting would be. She also gave me what were my first and most memorable pieces of advice.

"You will never be right again", she said. "You must learn quickly that it will be to your own advantage to give in to an argument and sometimes say sorry when you don't even know what you've done wrong." This made me smile as Dave often used to say when we argued, 'You've always got to be right haven't you?'

Annie had given me the date of the next Alzheimer's meeting and I thought it best to talk it over with Dave in the near future before becoming involved with, what I guessed, would be a mainly elderly group.

We had to acknowledge that we both needed support and advice, but at the same time I felt I had to warn him that there would be a lot of older people there. I would 'wing it' and mutter things like, 'They have a different type of dementia to you.' I would tell him, 'You won't be like that for years and anything could happen to either of us before then'.

I was desperate to protect him from thoughts of the future. I wanted to take all his fears away. Yet I know he was aware of his condition almost to the end of his life. He learned to take one day at a time.

The First Meeting

The meeting was exactly as I envisaged. Held in a church hall there were a lot of elderly people, a few in wheelchairs, with their carers chatting and having tea and biscuits. I could see the look of horror on Dave's face. You could not have come across a more compassionate man than him. In the past he had been involved with the elderly locally by helping run a Christmas party for pensioners, delivering harvest festival parcels, etc. He had also been involved with helping me in various charity works. Pre-diagnosis he would have swept into that room chatting to everyone, but standing in that church hall was like looking at a very bleak future. He had early onset dementia. Was this all that was on offer for younger people? Through that same support group we were soon to meet Sue and Richard. Sue became instrumental in organising pub lunches for younger people with dementia, which was a much better idea. We became, and still are, great friends.

Family Misunderstandings

Our daughters could always tell by my voice on the phone when things weren't right, and that must have been very frustrating for them. There were times when we were visiting them when there would be flare ups and I know they must have thought I wasn't handling things right. One Christmas at Jane's she overheard me being angry with Dave because I felt he was deliberately not co-operating when I was getting him ready for bed. I'm not proud of the times when I became impatient (and sometimes I did think Dave was being deliberately obstructive) but that's the nature of this evil illness. It plays tricks with the minds of the carer and the cared for. We shed quite a few tears that Christmas Eve. I had a lot of lessons to learn, but we ended up having a cuddle and moving on.

Similarly, when visiting Sue and family in Singapore, which we did in 2005, 2006 and 2007, there were a couple of frustrating incidents, but I know our hearts were in the right place and the girls only wanted what was best for both of us. I am proud of both of our daughters and their families and the support and love we've received from both of them over the years has been amazing.

Most books written about Alzheimer's dwell on the stages of the disease and how it takes away the person who is loved. I never felt as though I lost Dave just that occasionally someone else stepped inside his skin. He would become belligerent and then after a while I would get my Dave back. Although there were many aggressive incidents they often seemed funny in retrospect.

Action Plans

Support has always been there for me, whether it was from friends or family, but due to the concerns of both a plan of action was needed for difficult times. Sometimes neighbours could hear what was going on and would be quite worried so a house key was cut for both -Jean on one side of us and Ciara on the other - so they could come to our aid. Often before it got too bad I would ring Jean next door and she would come in to the house and that would be all we would need. A distraction, something to stop his train of thought. He was always happy to see Jean, well almost always, but sometimes chaos would reign.

Freedom Walks

Having showered and dressed Dave in the morning (he had lost those skills about five years into his illness) and given him and his breakfast he was ready to go out 'NOW'. Dave used to go for walks alone. Once he had begun to wander and road safety became an issue I knew the importance of getting him out and keeping him stimulated every day.

His frustration meant he wasn't prepared to wait for me to get dressed and this resulted in him kicking and banging on the glass door to get out. Sometimes, fearing the glass would break, I would open the door and let him go out while I got my shoes on. Then he would be off straight into the middle of the road, arms waving like a windmill shouting, 'I'm free, I'm free!'

This is when Jean next door would help out. Prior to this running off he used to have what the family called bagatelle walks where he would wander away from our road and friends and neighbours would turn him around and point him back in the right direction. I can laugh about it now but sometimes my heart would be in my mouth as I drove around looking for him.

Dave and the Policeman

The worst time was when he had been gone for three hours. Four friends in cars went looking for him, to no avail. So I made the decision to call the police. Never having dialled 999 before I was assured by the operator that I had done the right thing as he was considered a vulnerable adult.

I was in the process of giving a description of him when a car stopped outside. A friend had seen him from her kitchen window walking along a country, but busy, main road. She said that as she approached him he was having a conversation with a lady who had stopped her car and was no doubt telling him to walk on the footpath.

A police car pulled up at the same time and by the time we got Dave into the house the policeman was already sitting on the couch ready to take more details. I tried to point out how running off was dangerous and pointing to the policeman told Dave how worried everyone had been.

'Are you really a policeman?' he asked.

When the policeman said that he was, Dave saluted him, saying 'Attention!'

The policeman responded by smartly saluting back to him. This then became one of Dave's many sayings when greeting people, abbreviated to 'TENSHUN!' And people couldn't help but respond.

A particular incident comes to mind when I was desperately trying to calm him down. Sometimes the aggression would go on for a couple of hours or more and he would become so distressed. He would always repeat the same things, 'Why do you do this?' or 'Everything was happy before, why did you start it?' I usually had no idea what it was about other than his frustration about something. Sometimes it would be because I was tired and irritable and he may have picked up on that.

Whatever it was on this particular night it was getting out of control and I was getting frightened and blood pressure was rising. He was physically manhandling me near the bedroom window and I knew drastic measures were needed. Dave had always been aware of his condition and I could often talk him through things. I had an Aunt Betty who had recently been sectioned under the Mental Health Act and he understood this. In desperation, I begged him, 'Stop this now or I will have to call for help, Dave, and *this will* mean the police getting involved and you possibly being sectioned. Then, I will have no say on what will happen to you.'

By this time he was lying on his back on the bed and I thought this had done the trick, but no, 'HELP! HELP! POLICE!' he kept shouting. Goodness knows what anyone walking past would think. I'm sure there are experts in dementia who would disagree with the way I handled this but much as I valued all the training courses I did at the Carer's Centre, there are some situations which no amount of training can prepare you for.

Often after an incident like this he would cry himself to sleep and I would sit at the top of the stairs exhausted and heartbroken. I would want to wake him and tell him everything was alright but daren't in case the mood was still on him, and I would sleep in the other room. When he woke next morning and I went in to him he always looked subdued and almost frightened. It was important to both of us that I reassured him everything was alright and that if he did remember anything, he knew it was the illness and that he wasn't a bad person.

It was also important to apologise to him if I felt I hadn't handled the situation very well. 'Onward and upward', I would say and Dave would often sing, 'Always look on the bright side…'

Healthy Lifestyles

As Dave was aware of his condition and in fear of it, I felt we needed to be doing everything we could and not just sit waiting for the worse to happen. So we proceeded with omega fish oil, cranberry juice, plenty of fresh fruit and a general health diet. Exercise and fresh air were also very important but, because I have limited mobility when walking this is where our friends came to the rescue.

The Bowling Team

Dave absolutely loved bowling. It was also one of the first activities that showed there was a big problem. He belonged to our local club team and one summer evening he came home really distressed. He couldn't explain what had happened other than he felt as though the bowl was stuck to his hand and time had stood still. He could hear and see people but couldn't move.

The next day I met Terry, a team member, who asked how Dave was. He tried to explain what had happened but said they were all concerned as Dave didn't seem to be with them at all but just smiled at them and finally dropped the bowl. The whole bowling issue became a nightmare .Desperate to continue playing he asked me to mark the side of his bowl with something (we used nail polish) so he would know if he was playing finger or thumb.

Gradually he became worse but I'm ever grateful to the team who, when they knew they had won, put him on last so he felt part of the team. Our friend Joe said they always explained the situation to the opposing members and it was usually accepted with good grace. The club steward Tom said that only once was it challenged by a man from a visiting team who said, when told Dave had Alzheimer's, 'Well he shouldn't be playing then.'

'Well I hope you never get it', said Tom. This was probably the only time we had a negative response to anything. Joe and Arthur continued to practise with him when he was no longer part of the team.

Golf

Golf was another of Dave's hobbies. He was a member of a nine-hole golf course which belonged to a priests' seminary. The problem was it didn't allow guest members and after a couple of weeks of driving him there and walking the course with him I knew I wasn't physically able to continue doing this. I wrote to the secretary of the club and explained the situation and was given written permission for him always to be accompanied. This we put on a card on his golf bag so if the grounds man approached there wouldn't be a problem.

Cooperation again, which meant he was still in the loop with his good old mates. Our brother-in-law Paul was already a member of the club and would come and take him there, and then on for a pub lunch. Tom also used to take Dave to play golf or on walks. Then there was good old Jim who had never played golf regularly and after a few games damaged his shoulder. Every time he placed the ball on the tee it would be gone when he got his club out. They finally teed off and when they got to the next hole he noticed an odd shaped bulge in Dave's pocket. Yes, you've guessed it; Dave had three balls in his pocket! He didn't mind having a good laugh about it. He spent a lot of time laughing at himself in the early days in fact he was renowned for his sense of humour.

Noel, became a real golfing buddy who gave us cause for many a laugh. Noel had tunnel vision so it was thought it would be beneficial to both of them *to* play together. Noel would help Dave select his club and when Noel took a shot Dave would watch out for where it went. So Noel would take his shot, turn to ask Dave where it had gone, only to find him staring over the course miles away. 'Forgot to look', he would say. They lost a lot of balls that way and it took a long time to play for nine holes, but they did plenty of laughing afterwards while enjoying another pub lunch.

Once, when a different Consultant replaced Doctor Frances temporarily, he engaged with Dave in easy conversation. On asking how Dave was he got the usual, 'Fine, really great'. Asked what he had been doing lately he pondered for a while and then looked to me. I never liked to prompt him unless he looked to me for help. I reminded Dave of the game of golf the day before.

'You play golf?' 'Doctor said looking at me incredulously.

'Yes', said Dave looking at him proudly.

The doctor asked a few more questions regarding golf. 'How many holes do you play, do you have a handicap?

All the time the three of us were looking at one another in a puzzled manner. The Doctor because he couldn't believe what he was hearing. Dave because he didn't' know what the big deal was and as for me... I was squirming in my seat trying to indicate to the doctor that friends who took him were, without patronising Dave, letting him think he was playing the game.

Every time the doctor looked at me I would say something like, 'We have very good friends' or, 'It's a small fortune in lost golf balls'. At one point when the doctor looked at me amazed I thought of giving him a wink to let him know it wasn't a serious game and then I thought 'Oh my God, he might think I'm coming on to him'. At my age and as if there weren't enough problems to contend with!

Shortly after this I started doing my 'Caring With Confidence' course at the Carer's Centre. During the course we watched some filmed interviews with clients and carers. It was sometimes hard to know who was the client and who was the carer which made me realise how plausible people with dementia can be.

Did that Doctor really think Dave was playing a regular game of golf? Or was he so used to dealing with situations like this that he just rolled with it?

Getting Lost

Dave's love of walking and bird watching meant living near Carr Mill Dam was ideal for him in the early days, as he only had to walk to the bottom of the road , turn right and he would come to the footpath leading to the Dam. From there it was a circular walk on good footpaths where he was safe. There was often a fishing match on and Dave would often try and engage in conversation with the men involved. Some would be quite taciturn in their replies but most would respond.

I think the way people respond tells you whether they have had similar problems in their life. Walking around the Dam became impossible for me, yet knowing how much Dave loved it I decided that until something happened to worry me I had to let him have his independence.

Sure enough the day came when he didn't come home in the usual time. Instead of staying on the circular route he had gone under a bridge onto another foot path and walked in the opposite direction towards Haydock.

Having got there he lost his way and followed the road sign for St Helens. Once into St Helens Town centre he was able to find the road leading to Billinge, and so he continued to make his way home, even managing to get on a bus despite having no money with him.

His walk that day took him ten miles and he arrived home exhausted, parched and extremely agitated. I had been worried sick and had friends looking everywhere for him. Our friend Marj had been walking around Carr Mill Dam describing him to people and giving her phone number to the men who were fishing (I think she was disappointed when no one rang!).

We did some crying that day and we also made a decision that he should never walk on his own again. Time to accept a little more help from friends and family. So the walks continued as Pat and Arth, Howard and Marie would regularly take him on familiar routes over the fields via local footpaths and I would enjoy the respite.

Maintaining skills

Apart from a regime of fresh air and exercise I had been attempting to help Dave maintain his literacy skills and this he did with enthusiasm. (I treasure the five exercise books he completed). Every morning after breakfast I would get out his book, pen, some photos and maybe some literature about a holiday we might have had recently.

Before developing Alzheimer's Dave read three books a week and did a daily crossword. Within three years or so his literacy skills were failing him so it seemed important to replace them with something positive. Sometimes I would write some text for him to copy, whilst on other days he would feel more confident and be able to write freely about *a* holiday or a visit to the family. There were times when he struggled, became frustrated and then got upset calling himself stupid.

At times like this, sitting him down and trying to explain in simple terms that it was his illness stopping him from doing these things seemed to help. Explaining that his brain was unable to work things out like it used to I would say, 'You wouldn't call a person in a wheel chair stupid if their limbs wouldn't work, or ask them not to be silly and get up and walk'.

'No', he would reply.

'Then why call yourself silly or stupid because you have a condition of the brain which is stopping you doing thing? Let's think positively about the things we can do.'

It almost always worked.

If he told me he loved me and gave me one of his incredible smiles we would both feel better. He was always telling me he loved me. Of course it wasn't always that simple and I had to try and judge his mood. When I hadn't got it right and he went into a frustrated rage my inside would be churning. I was saying these things but my heart was breaking for all the losses he had to endure and I suppose I just wanted to make it go away.

Nobody gives out manuals as to how to deal with Alzheimer's. Courses at the Carer's Centre were extremely helpful but everyone is different and every carer is different. I like to think Dave and I were a team, and so did he. Consequently right to the end we talked things through and more often than not ended with Dave singing, you've guessed it, 'Always Look On The Bright Side Of life'.

Later life Memory Services

Dave's consultant decided that he should attend an assessment centre every Friday for ten weeks, organised by the 'Later Life Memory Services' (a much better title than The Old Age Psychiatric Unit, which was its previous title). Over this period of time, using 'Person Centred Dementia Care', there would be art therapy, games, reminiscence discussions plus what was to become the love of Dave's life, music and dancing. Prior to this illness Dave had been quite the introvert when it came to music; always last up on the dance floor at parties. Now I tended to worry if they played the music too loud in Tesco!

He absolutely loved these sessions which were staffed by trained dementia carers. At the end of the ten weeks it was recommended that Dave attend a day centre a few miles away, to stimulate him and give me respite. This had to be handled carefully. Once again I knew most clients would be elderly and infirm but there was nowhere for younger people with early onset dementia. We made an appointment to visit. I was impressed with how light and airy the building was, nice dining room, lovely lounges etc. but the grip Dave had on my fingers spoke volumes. He did warm to the staff who were extremely friendly, and with promises of him being able to help in the garden, we left on a positive note and he started going there.

Promises were kept and Dave was assigned a key worker who took him to buy plants, helped him to whitewash a garden wall and maintain some garden skills. However, after a few months, when waiting for the bus to pick him up, he started to become agitated, pleading with me not to send him and threatening to run off. Eventually I realised that it was the bus going all-around the world to pick people up that was the problem. So I decided to start taking him myself.

On arrival I could see, as I watched them helping elderly and infirm clients into the centre, why Dave wasn't settled. To have to witness people being spoon fed and helped to the bathroom was like Dave looking at his future. Driving him there and collecting him wasn't the answer.

'The doors are locked', he would say, 'I shouldn't be locked in. He told how an old lady had been rattling the door to get out, and telling everyone that she had her bag and keys'.

I know and trust that people were not left rattling doors all day by the staff but Dave was so in tune with his own condition that he watched out for this kind of thing. I was at the stage where I was desperate for a full day's break but the guilt was wearing me down. I simply couldn't accept that although I knew the importance of having a break for my own sanity, being told he would be alright when I left him wasn't enough, What was the point in having respite if I was feeling anxious all day? This was only the beginning of my quest for a place that catered for younger people with dementia and by now it was three years since Dave was diagnosed.   Contacting the hospital I asked if there was any possibility of Dave going back on Fridays to the Stewart Day Hospital, but was told that it was only for assessment. I asked if they could make allowances and let him continue to attend, even though he had already been assessed.   I was told that the sessions were only for people awaiting assessment and   there was a waiting list for them. I was clutching at straws; of course he couldn't remain in the Assessment Centre. So why was Dave happier there? In my opinion, a smaller number of clients and highly trained staff which of course meant more person centred care.

Chapter 7

THE QUEST FOR DAY CARE

Deciding to try another place nearer home for day care I was assured that Dave would be in the company of a couple of other younger people who had early onset dementia, but it was a similar situation. Too few staff with a heavy work load meant that Dave was left to his own devices until resident staff were bathed, fed etc.

One day, having gone on a day trip, I received a call on my mobile asking if I could come to the Home as Dave was extremely agitated. The fact that I was in Cheshire and had travelled there by coach meant I couldn't get there until late afternoon. I spoke to Dave on the phone and reassured him that I wouldn't be very long and then spoke to a carer asking, as it was such a sunny day, if he could be taken into the garden. I was told there weren't enough staff to enable them to do this. I was now feeling more guilt. Should I have gone on the day out?

I was always advised to view a care home without an appointment so when I made a decision to have a holiday break for a few days I did just that. I arrived unannounced and the receptionist rang for a carer to show me around a particular place which had a unit for Elderly Mentally Impaired. Dave had to be placed where there was such a unit as the risk of him walking out was too great. The carer walked ahead of me opening a succession of doors until we got to the unit. I could hear the noise of the clients from outside.

'It's alright here', she said, 'otherwise I wouldn't have been here all these years'.

When we got inside I felt heartsick.

'They're a bit noisy today', she said. 'We've sponged 'em all down because it's hot'.

The sight that greeted me was not pleasant. There was a man shouting and rocking his wheelchair, somebody crying and a lady, obviously disabled, crawling on the floor with her nightdress around her waist and incontinence pants on show. My eyes were drawn to the office in the corner where one member of staff was sitting at the desk, one on the desk, and two others were just leaning. Maybe they were having a meeting, I wondered! All I know is that I couldn't wait to get out of there.

Eventually I did find a suitable care home. Although the residents were once again very elderly, Dave seemed to click with the staff so I booked him into there for five days. Always worried that he would feel abandoned I arranged for friends and family to visit him each day. When I rang to see how he was on the first day I was told that he had been taken to the local social club next door where he had been made most welcome by the regulars. Word was passed around and each day his visitors took him there. It was a club where Dave could watch the locals play snooker and I was told that one day a man walked in and said, 'Hello there Dave. Here again and in my seat but that's o.k. You're welcome'. How lovely was that? Those regulars will never know what that meant to me.

Dave's Consultant then contacted me to say Dave would be accepted in a care home for younger people with dementia. Although still reluctant to go, as he really didn't see why I needed a rest, he did settle there more than he had anywhere else. After a while we decided to try an overnight stay and eventually some respite care while I had a mid-week holiday break. This care home believed in looking at their clients individually not just at the condition which meant using person centred care. I made sure Dave had his 'Who Me' book with him, which gave a brief history of Dave's life, including photos. He also had another album created by our grandchildren. This had more recent photos of all the family and grandchildren on holidays, on his last birthday and other events including funny captions written by the grandchildren. This gave carers another insight into Dave's family life. He became very fond of the carers there but seemed reluctant to integrate with other clients. which was understandable as not all were able to communicate. He did love it when there was music and dancing going on or musical entertainment of any kind.

However after about a year there a safeguarding alert was raised by social services and an investigation had to take place.

When I went to collect him one Sunday I noticed he had a graze/bruise on his forehead on the same spot where he'd had one the week before. I wasn't suspecting anything sinister but wondered whether there was something in his room that he was banging his head on. He could barely hold his head up he was so drowsy and he was drooling. I asked what medication he'd had and was told that he'd had none, by the nurse in charge. I told her that I had received a phone call the previous evening asking where Dave's Diazepam was and that I had informed them that it should be in their medicine trolley, but they disputed whether I had ever left it with them. If he hadn't had anything that day I asked what he'd been given the night before and was told that they didn't know. I just wanted to get him home and I needed the support of a carer to get him to the car. On arriving home it was impossible to get him out of the car on my own so I enlisted Jean's help. Once out of the car he was reeling all over the front lawn and speaking incoherently to Jean. I voiced my concerns to Dave's CPN (Community Psychiatric Nurse) Jeanette who, after spending some time talking to him herself, felt something just wasn't right. Later the same day she rang me and suggested that she 'flag this up' with social services for vulnerable adults and I agreed. When the investigation was complete social services recorded that the bruises could have been caused by a fall, unobserved , un-witnessed so unsubstantiated. Regarding the medication query, the Social Worker checked all case notes and found no misreporting of drug administration. So unsubstantiated again, safe guarding closed and no further action taken. While the investigation was going on I was offered another place for Dave elsewhere offering similar care for early onset dementia. I opted for one in Liverpool as it was a more straightforward journey. It was also in Kirkdale where Dave was born and lived until he married me in 1963. It was called Kavanagh Place.

Once the decision was made one of the senior members of staff, Craig, came out to see us with a carer named Sara. Little did I know then what a major part he would play in the the rest of Dave's life. He did an assessment of Dave and I don't know whether it was getting back to that scouse accent and Liverpool humour but they got on so well with Dave that we asked if we could view Kavanagh place as soon as possible. It was with trepidation and that old shadow of guilt that I went to view another care home; but I needn't have worried. The staff on every unit were so friendly and Martin, the manager, quietly reassuring and confident that they could meet Dave's needs.

We were given a tour of the place which was only three years old and had the latest equipment, a sensory room and three smaller lounges, rather than that stereotypical large lounge with its circle of chairs. We were introduced to all staff, including those in kitchen and laundry, who were obviously very involved with the clients. There was a training room where staff from other care homes could receive training, which reassured me that their own staff would be fully trained.

Dave was behaving as though he has known everyone all his life. I really do think that the Liverpool accent made all the difference. When we were in the lift as Craig was escorting us out he asked us if we had any questions. I had none.

'We've one for you haven't we Dave?' said our friend Pat. 'Which football team do you support, Liverpool or Everton?.

Craig laughed and said to Dave, 'What are you Dave, a blue or a red?'

Dave replied, 'Blue'. He had been a lifelong Liverpool supporter and now in his confusion he thought he was a blue.

We were asked to continue Dave's care at the previous care home but I asked if we could stay put as Dave was so well settled. It was worth the longer journey and thank goodness this was agreed by The Community Health Care Team. He still sometimes had some reluctance and he would get upset when taking him there. The difference was, I was invited to have a cup of coffee and wait while they placated him and then he would say good bye happily. When I returned for him, to whoops of joy and hip hip hurray, he didn't want to pull and push me out of the place as he had done in other places. He would ask me to sit down with him, and hold hands and ask if I wanted a cup of tea. That spoke volumes to me.

Chapter 8

SOCIAL LIFE

Once Dave was established in Kavanagh place I could accept the fact that, apart from short walks with friends, we would be inseparable during the week. I still took him over to the club for his Friday night pint, which had become shandy, as just a small amount of alcohol would have a bad effect on Dave. I gave him the right price in pounds and asked friends not to buy him anymore. I also had a word with the bar staff so that no one would pity him and buy him a drink.

The important thing was he was still socialising with his old friends. We still went out with friends and to friends' homes for meals but sometimes it was difficult in public. I was sad for him when his 'Christmas night out' around Liverpool with friends had to stop, but it became too risky as he could easily have got lost in a crowded city. I knew my friends worried about their own husbands going on this jaunt. These men have been our friends for forty odd years, bless 'em but they still think they are young lads about town on that night. The offers of, 'I'll look after him Joan', had to be met with a grateful refusal as they always lost one another but usually met up at the train station.

It was arranged that we should have a carer from Crossroads, a charity based care agency, one afternoon a week. I chose to have a Friday afternoon so I could catch up on house work and shopping so my weekend respite would mean it was 'me' time. We had two carers, Marie and Doreen, on alternate Fridays. Marie would either stay home with him and sometimes do reminiscence activities, or maybe take him out for tea and cakes, usually to the Garden Centre.

Doreen, who was with him for a few years, revelled in his love of music .The louder the better. She usually took him for walks around Taylor Park where they fed the ducks, and then to a café on the way home for toasted teacakes. This was so good for Dave as he was still physically fit. If I got home before them and was unloading shopping from the car I would hear the music coming from Doreen's car as it came around the corner, both of them singing away usually to Elvis, but often Dave would be giving a rendition of 'Always Look On The Bright side'.

Sadly for Doreen she had to experience the aggressive side of Dave before he eventually went into residential care.

I was driving into town one day when my mobile rang. It was Doreen asking if I could come home quickly as Dave was in a rage and she didn't know what had triggered it. When I got home he was sitting in the dining room looking furious and refusing to speak to me. I put some relaxing music on and Doreen and I had a coffee whilst Dave drifted off to sleep. Unfortunately this incident happened a couple of times and each time she would have to ring for me, culminating in him really frightening her by pulling at the scarf around her neck.

From then on it was agreed that I should stay home, sometimes getting on with some work and other times just joining in their company as they danced and sang. We both knew that Dave was getting worse and there would come a time when residential care was going to have to be considered, but for the time being he still loved Doreen.

Another carer we had for a time was Aaron who was a natural with Dave and took him on walks or to a local pub to watch a game of pool or sport on T.V. They made an unlikely pair as they ambled around Billinge and people often said to me, 'I saw Dave and his grandson going for a walk today'.

Aaron was accepted for nurse training at university so our loss was the nursing profession's gain. He even remembered Dave's 70th birthday party and called in with a card for him.

On other days we continued with our picnics, visiting the Martin Mere bird sanctuary and the cinema where, in the winter, we used to sneak hot pies and sausage rolls in for a late lunch as eating out had become a bit of a problem. So to all those patrons of cineworld whose mouths were watering at the delicious smell of hot pies and sausage rolls and to the management of course, I apologise.

Also for Dave's interruption of the film as he joined in the dialogue. 'What's your name'? was asked in one film.

'David, David Crank', he replied in a very loud manner.

Even worse would be when he decided to repeat a swear word really loudly. This often happened when we went along with friends, culminating in them stifling their laughter. I don't think he could always follow films but it was the social event that was important to him. It was worth the effort of springing that cinema seat up and down several times before I finally got him to sit down. We were the pre-film entertainment!

The bird sanctuary was great, but the only drawback was when we had walked around and seen most of the birds he would get tired and say, 'Are we going now?'

There was a room used for educational purposes where it was ok to have picnic lunches, so sometimes we would go there and look at the children's art work from visiting schools. The only problem was that if a school party came in he would want to approach them and he had such a caring friendly manner that children would often respond. Of course I understood that this was a problem for the staff who were responsible for their welfare.

I would often approach staff and explain the situation and it was surprising how many people had experience of this condition with family or friends. However, we didn't stay around long if a party of children did arrive as it would have been chaotic if Dave started a game of chase!

Don't forget Dave had been the Father Christmas of Billinge for years, driven around on a tractor before the opening of the school Christmas Fayre.

Knowsley Safari Park :
The Safari Park was a real favourite and for many years we had been renewing our annual pass. As soon as we went through the gates and started on the route it was as if we were in another world whatever the season. The first view was usually the Deer which Dave would rave about but even the pheasant, Emu and Ostrich were greeted with the same enthusiasm. The odd Pigeon that had flown in was also acknowledged and also the scenery. Anyone would have thought we had never seen trees and grass before.

The Tiger   enclosure had large platforms for viewing them but they often were hidden from view. I found it most frustrating when the Tigers were in full view on the platforms but, because of Dave's diminishing spatial awareness, I couldn't get him to see them.

'Yes, I'm looking', he would say whilst looking the opposite way. To hold his chin and try and turn his head didn't work as he would angrily repeat, 'I can see them'.

It was me who was becoming frustrated, as I so badly wanted him to see them. Once again I had to repeat to myself the word, 'acceptance'. He couldn't always see everything but he was having a nice day.

The Lion enclosure was a firm favourite of both of us, especially when there were cubs. We would drive through slowly trying to count the pride and their cubs. We had been doing this for about seven years or so, until the day Dave tried to get out of the car.

Before entering the safari route I had tried to get Dave to remove his jacket as it was very warm but he refused. I tried to explain that once we were in the enclosure he wouldn't be able to take it off, but to no avail. Within a few yards he was hot and struggling to undo his seat belt. Even with the air conditioning on we were both in a bit of a state. He then struggled to open the door. The air was blue and to any observers it must have looked like a domestic as we wrestled.

'Look, there are Lions everywhere. This is very dangerous', I said.

'Don't be (bleep bleep) silly', he said.

By this time he was raging and was becoming very aggressive as he struggled. He was desperate to get out of the car and had no sense of danger. There was a Park Ranger in his safari jeep up ahead so I thought a blast on my car horn would do the trick. I envisaged a scene where it would turn from what looked like a domestic, to a full scale brawl with the Park Ranger, so

I ignored the traffic sign which stated the speed limit in the enclosure was 5mph and put my foot down. As I was weaving my way through other traffic I could hear the Ranger on his loud hailer, 'Madam there is a speed limit in this enclosure, Will you slow down please'.

My usual conservative driving manner was compromised by the need to escape from Lions, and another time by Dave's need of a toilet – another occasion when he tried to get out of the car. Once we got out of the enclosure and it was safe to stop and remove his jacket he was fine.

'There you are, see. That's all I wanted', he said, completely unaware that my nerves were in shreds. We continued to visit the safari park but gave the Lions a miss from that day.

Then we became a threesome with my lovely Aunt Betty joining us on safari park visits. When she developed dementia her son Barry and family asked her to move in with them as it was thought she was becoming a danger to herself. Dave and I had already been regular Sunday afternoon visitors to the family and after dinner had some really good old sing-a-longs with a bit of dancing thrown in. However, Barry drew the line at being Dave's dance partner.

Being able to take Betty on a Tuesday afternoon would hopefully be a change for everyone. We had bought Betty a season ticket for the safari Park for her 80th birthday. The first time we went there she said, 'Do you know, of all the years I lived in Liverpool I've never been here.'

Dave would reply, 'Haven't you? Oh! You are really going to love it'.

This conversation was to be repeated every Tuesday afternoon. It was like Groundhog Day but, actually having the two of them for company was easier than just Dave on his own.

The monkeys were the most amusing and going the car friendly route meant we could park up and watch their antics, or they would watch us. I could almost imagine them saying, 'Well look who's here again. It's that Joan, Dave and Betty'. When we returned home we would have our meal together and then Barry would come and take her home.

Chapter 9

TRAVELLING TO SEE CHILDREN AND

GRANDCHILDREN

It was important that, although our immediate family lived so far away, we maintained regular close contacts and visits as I had a dread of Dave forgetting who they were. We managed to get out to Singapore three times and on our return home he once wrote in his daily writing practice book, 'When we came down the elevator at the airport I could see Sue and the children with a big welcome banner waiting for us. I will never forget that.'

Flying so far wasn't easy, even with assisted travel, but oh so worth it. Handling those trays of food meant me cutting up Dave's food, getting rid of all foil lids then swapping trays. Going to the toilet, I would leave the door partially open asking the stewardess to explain to other passengers why I needed to do this and then I could manage if Dave needed help with his clothing.

The worse thing that happened was when we changed planes at Dubai and we had to go through a security check within the airport. He was asked to remove his shoes and there was nowhere to sit down whilst doing this. We were both feeling extremely tired and the officials looked on while we struggled. Fortunately we were travelling with our friends who were able to support us and when we got through security found a chair for him to sit down and get the shoes back on. There was the language barrier, I know, but the unsmiling security staff just stared as we tried to show by gestures that we had a problem.

Dementia training classes for stewards and all airport staff would be a major help. Perhaps the Alzheimer's Society's initiative of Dementia Friends and Dementia Champions, where people with some knowledge are prepared to talk to groups about dementia would be helpful. Going through security has always been particularly problematic for me.

The crew on planes were always helpful and attentive. I remember once when returning home a fellow passenger told us that Sir Bobby Charlton was in first class and could be seen through the partition curtain stood at the bar. 'I'm off to see him', said Dave and no amount of pleading stopped him. I followed looking for a steward to help but before I could do anything Dave had gone into first class, shaken hands with Sir Bobby and was on his way back towards me.

'What a lovely fella Bobby is', He said to a fellow passenger.

'Sir Bobby', said the passenger.

'He's always been Bobby to me and always will be', said Dave.

The time spent in Singapore was precious as we got to spend a lot of quality time with Sue, Wayne and our grandchildren. Matt the eldest would patiently listen to his granddad and try to understand him. Sophie is a great mimic and would have him laughing as she tried out all her different accents and Jessica the youngest was just delighted to have him pick her up from school.

Swimming was Dave's favourite pastime there and, as they had their own pool, there were no worries regarding changing rooms. It was out of our bedroom and straight into the pool. There was a game we played called Marco Polo where one person kept their eyes shut while the others swam around shouting Marco.

The person with eyes closed would swim towards anyone and shout, 'Polo'. It was impossible for Dave to understand this so he would shout words like loco, cocoa or poco, anything but polo and have the children in tears with laughter. Each time they tried to get him to say it he would nod, smiling away, but you know I swear he was doing it on purpose. He could always laugh at himself.

They had a live-in helper called Carrie as was customary out there. She was very fond of Dave, called him granddad and was forever offering him bananas saying they were good for his health. If Dave went to walk outside the gates alongside a field to look for birds she would stand outside and just watch that he didn't go too far. I asked her if she had known anyone with Alzheimer's disease before and she said the word wasn't used in the Philippines where it was just called old persons' disease.

Being in Singapore meant that we could also do the things that make grandparents proud, such as going to netball matches to watch how athletic Sophie and Jessica were and swimming lessons and galas in Olympic size swimming pools. Saturday mornings when we cheered on Matthew playing rugby (yes, in that tropical heat), it wasn't just Dave that sometimes cheered on the wrong child.

When I look back I'm amazed at just how much travelling we did from Singapore to Phuket and Lankawi in Malaysia, where we took a boat trip and the owner threw a bucket of fish into the river and the mountain eagles came down to feed. I will never forget the expression on Dave's face as they all swooped around us.

Kuala Lumpur was where I made the mistake of thinking we could walk to the twin towers from our hotel. Dave got hot and tired, sat down on the floor furious with me and I called a taxi. When it came to getting into the taxi all coordination had gone and he sat on the floor instead of the seat swearing profusely. The taxi driver couldn't understand why he was so angry. That day I learned never to just wander, but to always take an organised tour.

Much as we loved going out to see them I was so grateful when they came back to England and settled in Guildford a couple of years ago. It was becoming more and more important to have regular contact, so that when we went down south or they came up north there was more of a chance he would still recognise his grandchildren.

Going down to Hampshire to Jane, Paul and the grandchildren Amelia (Millie) and Annie (not forgetting the dog Pippin) was also not without problems but again so worth it.

Once again planning and the help of friends made it possible. We always went by train so to get to the station meant enlisting the help of one of our friends as they understood getting Dave into a car could be difficult .Also I was more relaxed with friends as I never knew what kind of a conversation Dave would strike up with a taxi driver. Among family and friends I encouraged Dave to join in conversations and they were very patient giving him time to think but, with strangers I did get a bit stressed.

Once again I would organise assisted travel with the rail company. Watching for our coach number as the train came in, then getting Dave and luggage on was something I dreaded. When the train did come in people on the platform surged towards the doors but, with a guard to assist us, I didn't worry about not getting on before the train pulled out and also the guard would get the luggage on for me.   Except for once, when leaving Wigan Northwest, a passenger called to me, 'Where do you want this case love?'. The guard had asked him to take the case for him. It only happened once though.

Wheelchairs, crutches and walking sticks are visible and given space but Alzheimer's disease is not a visible illness and certainly not in a healthy and handsome man in his sixties. Dave carried a card explaining his illness and I also carried one, but to flash my card whilst being jostled would have come across as sarcastic as mine said,

'MY PARTNER HAS ALZHEIMERS DISEASE, THANK YOU SO MUCH FOR YOUR PATIENCE'.

I would also have lost both the card and Dave in the crush. The card does, however, work in shops.

We had to change trains at Wolverhampton for Basingstoke and I was always so relieved to find a guard waiting for us to make sure we got our connection. He would then see us onto the next train where I would heave a sigh of relief and then we would have our picnic lunch, with coffee in a flask, as going to the buffet car was not an option. Going to the toilet we had to be together to the amusement of any one standing near, but I learnt not to make eye contact with anyone while Dave said hello to everyone. In the toilet I would keep repeating to Dave, 'Please don't touch the buttons'. I had this dread of that door slowly sliding open.

Having reserved seats didn't always make a difference as if someone was in our seats they weren't always willing to move and once again I would have to try and explain Dave's disability discreetly. Once we had a lady who refused to cooperate even when I leaned over and quietly explained Dave's condition.

'I know all about Alzheimer's. My mother had it', she said 'but I'm not moving. My bags are at my feet and I have a bad back so I'm sorry'. All this in a very loud voice, and consequently Dave was becoming agitated.

There wasn't another seat in the coach other than the nearby one I wanted her to move to. Asking her if she would mind me leaving Dave sitting next to her while I went to ask the guard if he could   find me two seats together she looked horrified. 'Will he be alright?' she said.

At this point other passengers became involved, swapping seats so she wouldn't have to move far and moving her bag for her. I was so grateful they could see our predicament. The seats were reserved for that very reason so we could sit quietly together, and I'm sure that, confronted by a healthy looking man, the lady didn't realise how her elderly mother's dementia was not comparable with Dave's early onset dementia.

This is something other carers and I often discuss; how bizarre behaviour in our partners when they are disturbed can be so challenging to us, whereas until there is a crisis they appear so normal to others. The journey continued peacefully. Dave relaxed and so did I eventually and the lady in question carried on with her knitting. All was well with the world.

When we did arrive at our destination the sight of Jane and the children waiting made it so worthwhile and Dave would sit in the back of the car with Millie and Annie to discuss what we were going to do on this visit. They live in a cottage in a beautiful location off the beaten track with just a couple of cottages on either side. Opposite their front door is a common which meant plenty of room to run around with granddad without having to worry about traffic. There was also a wood nearby where we could walk the children and use the tree swings.

Millie, from a very early age, seemed aware of granddad's vulnerability and spent a lot of time listening patiently when he talked to her. Annie had communication difficulties from an early age and as a result had speech therapy. She once said to her mum, 'Granddad has problems with his words like I do'. Somehow she connected with Dave. I remember once when they arrived at our house she was so excited about a book she brought with her. 'Granddad', she said, 'You are going to love reading this book with me. It's about a giant who gets all his words muddled. Just like you do'. It was Roald Dahl's BFG book. I think Annie and Dave realised each other's problems.

Center Parcs was somewhere we visited a couple of times but on the second occasion I felt that we shouldn't hire bikes as Dave's coordination was getting worse. This was about five years after he was diagnosed. However, Jane and Paul thought it was worth giving it a try and they would be responsible for him. Paul checked that the bike seat was OK and told

Dave to leave it in the gear he had put it in. A practice ride around the car park and they were off. They were fine for a couple of days, but then on the third day I had decided to have a leisurely stroll and meet them later (my nerves wouldn't stand me joining them on the ride.)

It wasn't until much later I discovered that Dave had failed to apply the brakes and went careering into a group of elderly people out for a walk. Fortunately no one was hurt apart from Dave having a few scratches and, as Jane said, it was so worth it just to see the joy on his face.

It was at the swimming pools at Centre Parcs where the most fun (and frights) were had. Jane tried to point out the warning signs to him saying, 'Dad, look it says, go down the slide feet first'.

'OK,' he would say and then dive in head first. When he got to the bottom he would lie arms outstretched floating face down until Jane or Paul pulled him up. Had he perhaps forgotten what to do next?

There was a plunge slide with very deep water at the bottom, which had red and green lights and one could only go down on a green light. Paul made a sudden decision to go down and Dave immediately followed him giving everyone else a fright.

Playing around the smaller pools with Annie he would try to pick up somebody else's child going up or coming down the slides. If they had the same coloured swimwear as Annie he would go wading in, ignoring our cries telling him that it wasn't Annie. He was never left alone so one of us could always explain if he got any strange looks.

I have to confess that I took advantage of all this activity and spent a lot of time in the Jacuzzi chatting with other grandparents. Millie and Annie called the Jacuzzi 'Grandma Soup', as we all looked as though we were simmering away.

What wonderful times we had with our grandchildren on both sides of the world. Dave would say, 'Joan, aren't we so lucky?'

I would say, 'That's right Dave, 'Always Look on the Bright side'. He really was amazing.

Chapter 10

EXTENDED FAMILY AND FRIENDS

Dave's extended family had always been close and I'm sure they must have found it difficult as Dave's dementia progressed. He always saw Barbara and Derek regularly but, as Edward, his youngest brother, had moved back to Liverpool we only saw him on special occasions.

Moving Dave to a different care home enabled them to develop a closer relationship as Edward could visit him when he was in for weekend or holiday respite. Apparently Dave would greet him with, 'Here's our Eddie'.

With typical scouse humour the staff would say to me when I arrived to collect Dave, 'Our Eddie's been in'.

Derek was already in regular contact with Dave as they had both worked for RIDING FOR THE DISABLED in retirement. This was something Dave loved and we once went to an RDA Mini Olympic event in Yorkshire. Ella and I stood in the stands cheering as Derek and Dave carried the banner of our group. The sight of so many people challenged in different ways, some walking, some in wheelchairs made us so proud to be part of the event. It seemed Ironic that Dave was leading the group but would shortly be regarded as a person with special needs.

Sadly Dave had to retire from his voluntary work as he was unable to follow instructions regarding the safety of clients but Acorn farm, which was the base for RDA, became a place to visit for a long time to come. This simply meant a change of activity; Derek would arrive ready to take Dave for a walk or have a look around the garden to see if he could help Dave a little.

It must have been hard for all the family and friends in those days as I was attending courses at the Carers Centre regarding living with dementia and would be forever spreading my knowledge and expecting them to listen to my every word. As if I always got it right! Any printed hand-outs from the Carers' Centre would be duly handed around and expected to be read. One thing I couldn't control was the progression of his illness, but I could try and make sure we were all aware of any changes.

Going out to restaurants became stressful and Dave began to tire earlier in the evenings so our friends accommodated us by inviting us to lunch, or family would visit in the evening when we would play Dave's favourite music and even have a dance, which was Ella's job.

Our Sunday afternoon's with Barry and family continued almost to the end of Dave's life.

When it was Derek and Ella's golden wedding Anniversary they had a great family get- together. As Dave was losing his inhibitions more and more his greeting of Ella was quite flirtatious with a warm kiss on arrival and another one on departure. I think that was one of the most enjoyable occasions apart from the last one which was his seventieth birthday.

When we arrived at the party there were members of Ella's family whom we hadn't seen for years. Dave had been best man at their wedding and so they wanted the same wedding group for a photo. They were all duly put in position for the photo once they could get Dave to stand still and, once the photo was taken Dave proceeded to hug and kiss everyone. He then worked his way around the room greeting people, or being greeted by people, he hadn't seen for years with a look of amazement or extreme surprise on his face. He danced the night away and the evening culminated with a huge circle of family and friends singing 'You'll Never Walk Alone' and 'New York, New York'.

On leaving Dave proceeded to thank everyone for coming and telling them all what a brilliant night and wasn't it great of them all to put this night on for him.

I'm sure Derek and Ella didn't mind him stealing a little bit of their thunder that night and I know people found it hard to believe there was much wrong with him, particularly as he appeared to remember them. Sometimes I wondered if he was bluffing as this is something people with dementia are adept at doing.

Having asked his Consultant some time previously if the scan showed where the damage was I was told it was the frontal lobe. I recently read the following description of frontal temporal dementia in TELLING TALES ABOUT DEMENTIA edited by Lucy Whitman.

'At an early stage memory usually remains intact while personality and behaviour -
including social skills and the ability to empathise with others - may change radically.
Language skills may also become damaged. At a later stage symptoms are usually similar
to those of Alzheimer's disease. Frontal-temporal dementia may develop at any age,
but is more likely to affect people under 65'.

All the people I have met with dementia, and there have been so many over the years, are so different, but I still could never understand why Dave lost so many life skills so early; telling the time, literacy, numeracy, using cutlery, managing personal hygiene, etc and yet be able to go into social situations and greet people without hesitation.

Barbara and Paul were also regular visitors and Dave was always delighted to see his only sister, 'our Barb'. In the last year or so he would look at her and say, 'MAM' or, 'MUM'. We all somehow knew there was no confusion about who Barbara was as he would laugh when he said it. It was simply that he recognised the resemblance to his Mother.

Sometimes some of the carers from the support group would arrange a meal out and one night Barbara came with her son Stephen so I would be able to go. Getting out of the car one night on returning home I could hear Stephen's laughter from outside the house. Dave had been in great form dancing on his own, making his own words up to songs and trying to persuade Stephen to dance with him. Stephen said he would come with his mum to sit anytime as it was the best night out he'd had in ages.

On another occasion both sons came as I had some very heavy curtains that needed hanging. I went out for the carers' meal while they did this for me. The job was done when I returned and Andrew told me that Dave had been struggling to tell him that he had put the rail up a long time ago. I couldn't believe it. It was something I had totally forgotten about. Two years before he was diagnosed Dave had been struggling to put a new curtain rail up. He just hadn't been able to manage what would once have been such a simple job for him. He resorted to cutting the rail rendering it useless. He then tried to bind it with string and eventually abandoned it angrily. Boy, was the air blue that day!

He went out and bought another rail, refused to let me help, and so the struggle began again. Jean from next door came in and we enlisted the help of another neighbour. Eventually the job was completed but I could see Dave's distress, even though everything had been handled in the most diplomatic manner. When, a couple of years later I told our neighbour of Dave's diagnosis he immediately said, 'The Curtain rail, that explains it'. There we were nearly ten years later and

Dave had made a connection with the curtain rail, but he wouldn't have been able to tell you where he'd been that day or what he'd had for dinner that evening. Baffling!

Family gatherings meant so much to Dave and they didn't have to be happy occasions. Following a family funeral we had gone for lunch when I noticed Dave standing at the bar with his nieces and nephews. Having asked that no one buy him alcohol because of the adverse effect I could tell Dave was pulling faces behind my back to a chorus of 'Ah's. Later on sitting around a table having eaten Dave looked around the table and with a huge smile upon his face said, 'Hands up all those having a nice time?'

Everyone had to stifle their laughter as I said, 'Dave we are at a funeral'. But the time was coming when I would never again have to explain Dave's behaviour.

Friends can be almost as close as family and none so more than Jean and Ian who live next door and have done for 48 years. In the beginning they used to come up to paint and decorate (or so they said) and we were soon friends as well as neighbours. We had our children, returned to work and then came retirement. In all that time we had never had a cross word.

In the last few years their grandson Jake would knock on the back door to see if Dave was coming out to play, and if our car wasn't on the drive he would say to Jean, 'They must have gone to the Safari Park'.

He was a real little buddy to Dave and it just seemed so natural. Little did I know how much I would come to value this relationship.

After the initial shock of Dave's diagnosis Ian would always keep his eye on Dave when he attempted any DIY projects. He even rescued him off the roof once (more about that later). Jean was always there for me emotionally as I could escape there for a good cry when the frustration got too much. I've lost count of the times when she ran after Dave and they would come back up the road arms linked as she comforted him.

Very often Dave would suddenly become upset and I wouldn't be able to figure out what it was. If I hadn't got a plan for that day then we would try and work through it, but one particular day we had been invited to a 21st birthday party. I had offered to do a couple of dishes towards the catering and had been in the kitchen most of the morning. In retrospect I had not given him the attention he and most sufferers needed.

Suddenly I heard those dreaded words, 'I'M OFF', and the sound of the front door being kicked. I dropped everything and told him we would be going out very soon, but to no avail. Party or not, he wasn't going, yet he wanted me to go, as upset as he was.

He was adamant about this. I don't know whether he needed time alone or didn't want me to miss out on the party. Whatever the reason he wasn't open to persuasion. A quick phone call and in came 'Aunty Jean' to the rescue. She went upstairs to him, sat on the bed and cried with him, sensing his frustration. When she came down she said he was adamant that he wasn't going but he wanted me to go. It was an afternoon party and the last thing I felt like doing was going as I was so upset but I went to take the food and stay for a couple of hours.

Dave had a sleep, watched T.V. and Jean nipped in every 20 minutes or so to check he was alright or needed a drink. I rang her regularly for a report and she reassured me he was o.k. When I came home he was subdued but I knew that for once we had handled it right. He had needed some space. This was just one of the many, many occasions that I was rescued by my lovely neighbours.

Chapter 11

SOUTH AFRICA 2002

Having been to Australia for a wedding we decided to attend the wedding of our friends' son and his lovely Australian bride to be held in South Africa. This was in 2002, only weeks before Dave's formal diagnosis. Also it was a chance to do some touring and visit Kruger Park. We had already started investigations regarding Dave's difficulty with word finding and several other symptoms and when we got home after the holiday it was to find that a brain scan had been arranged.

We arrived in Cape town and that evening had dinner with the bride's family who had arrived from Australia. It was arranged that the few days preceding the wedding were to be spent touring in a bus. Both families got on so well as we visited beaches, crowded with puffins and seals, viewed Table Mountain, Robin Island and generally took in the sights. We also went to the top of Table Mountain in a chair lift. The view from up there was amazing.

Dave kept saying, 'I can't believe after geography lessons at school we are actually looking at Table Mountain'.

The only thing that blighted it was the worry of Dave losing his words and sometimes it came out like complete gibberish. At one point on the coach he started talking normally to one of the party when suddenly words literally failed him. The look of horror on his face panicked me and Toni's sister seemed to be looking to me for help. He clung on to my hand as we continued the tour, both of us frightened. I had no idea then that damaged speech was a symptom.

It was at the wedding reception that Dave's behaviour really started to change. I noticed he had become very loud and couldn't seem to settle in his seat. After several visits to the toilet, when he got lost every time, we enjoyed a delicious meal finishing with a desert intricately decorated with spun toffee. Dave picked his up by the toffee and began to swing it to and fro. 'What's this supposed to be?' he shouted.

There we were in one of the top hotels in the world and he was behaving like a lager lout.

'Who's that man over there with the bad comb-over?' he shouted, pointing to the man on a nearby table. When I tried to remonstrate with him he couldn't focus when trying to look at me.

Although there was champagne immediately after the wedding he'd had very little to drink. Not being a drinker myself I was able to observe him, but, although this was much earlier on in the day, I realised that perhaps it was the alcohol that was the cause. Returning to the table and finding Dave accepting a refill from the waiter I began to quietly plead with him not to drink anymore. 'Oh shut up', he said and when the speeches started he kept shouting out rude comments. Pat and Arth' assured me that this didn't spoil anything but I really didn't want Toni's family to think this was the real Dave.

After the reception we returned to the apartments and were invited in by the family for a nightcap. I was persuaded that Dave would be alright, but I asked him not to drink anymore. His alcohol intake for the whole day had not been that much but I was soon to discover that even a small amount would affect him greatly. I soon realised that he would only get worse and so persuaded him to come back to our own apartment where he continued to be just downright nasty to me.

Sitting there crying I told him I would have to cancel our tour of South Africa and see if we could we get a flight home the following day.

'You do that', he roared at me, pulling the duvet over him.

This was not my lovely husband Dave and I was so confused and frightened sitting there when he suddenly sat up arms outstretched. 'Help me Joan', he said. 'What's happening to me. I'm scared.'

We both cried ourselves to sleep after trying to reassure one another. Our hopes were pinned on some sort of solution from the professionals when we returned home.

We did continue our tour in a safari jeep, with the odd struggle with word finding, enjoying the awe inspiring scenery and wonderful sunsets. We stayed in Lodges and on an Ostrich farm (yes, Dave did saddle up and ride an ostrich) until we finally got to Kruger Park where we saw so many animals in the wild. Some nights we would sit around the camp fire enjoying a BBQ cooked by our guide and toasting marshmallows.

I remember Pat's son Robin, who had known Dave all of his life, asking me as we stood on the balcony of their apartment what I thought could be the cause of Dave's change in behaviour. By this time I had several theories of my own. 'I think it's a chemical imbalance of the brain', I said , 'and when we get home all his blood results will be back and they will be able to prescribe something to balance things out.'

Oh that it would be so simple!

Chapter 12

RUBY WEDDING AND THE QE2 CRUISE

Having finally got a diagnosis, we tried to live our lives as normally as possible. We continued with daily activities taking the 'if you don't use it, you lose it' attitude. Dave was prescribed Aricept, and although we knew it wasn't a cure but would only slow things down, psychologically it had a marked effect on him and he appeared to become more confident.

On the 31st August 2003 it was our Ruby wedding Anniversary, just one year after diagnosis We celebrated by having a wonderful party attended by all our family and friends in our local club. During the party surrounded by our daughters, sons in law and grandchildren, we were presented with flowers and Sue said a few words of congratulations.

I thanked everyone for coming, for their gifts but most of all for their support. I also told them we were doing well and I expected to see them all at our Golden wedding celebration. There were a few tears shed by guests. You know we almost made it. We were just 15 months short of our Golden wedding anniversary when Dave died.

To continue celebrating the year of our Ruby Anniversary we decided, literally, to push the boat out and go on the first cruise of our lives. It was to be on the QE2 on a cruise called South American Adventure calling at ports in Brazil, Uruguay, Falkland Islands, Senegal, Canaries and Madeira before arriving back in Southampton. The cruise was to last 31 days and was quite stormy at times but fortunately neither of us was sea sick.

I knew we might have some difficulty, so on the first night I quietly had a word with our waiter regarding Dave's condition and he agreed to only put out the cutlery he would need for each course. He also quite casually would recommend certain dishes so that Dave wouldn't be overwhelmed with choice or struggle to read the menu. Meals became a pleasure.

Lifeboat Drill was something I hadn't thought about and although well organised it seemed a bit manic to Dave and I. Finding our way around the ship was as hard for me as it was for Dave for the first few days. Some friends had bought us radio transmitters so we could contact each other on the ship, but on trying them out at home between the garden and the house I couldn't get Dave to press the button when talking, so he would end up shouting from the bottom of the garden. We had some laughs trying though.

On one of the formal evenings we went to the Captains cocktail party where there was a bit of confusion greeting people. In the officer's line-up Dave wanted to shake hands with whoever he pleased in whatever order he wanted, but this was taken in good humour and all went well.

That is until we joined some fellow guests who were discussing health issues in old age. One of the men put two fingers to his head as though cocking a gun and said, 'I know one thing as I get older if ever I get Alzheimer's disease I want a gun putting to my head'.

Dave gripped my hand under the table. What a sweeping statement to make. I wanted to say to that man, 'It's not that bad. Look at us cruising around South America . We've still a lot of living to do'. How controversial that would have been for cocktail party chit chat.

After we left to go to the restaurant we had a bit of a giggle as to what their faces would have been like had I said any of those things. Normally open and up front regarding Dave's condition this was not a time to open up as it would have spoiled the evening for the other guests. The ship was so big we never saw them again and who knows if someone else in that company might have been in the same situation as us.

The weather was so rough (force 11 gale) when we reached the Falkland Islands that we were unable to go ashore at Port Stanley. This was a bitter disappointment to many as the QE2 had been deployed during the Falklands war in 1982. She had carried the main British Land Fighting Force to the Falklands before the South Atlantic winter closed in, which would have made the taking of the Falklands impossible. What I found most heart rending was the fact that along with the former governor of the Falklands, who was delivering lectures about the war on days at sea, there were parents of soldiers from the ship Sir Galahad, who had lost their lives during the Argentina/Falkland Islands war of 1982.

Dave had been most interested in these talks and all this information. The Sir Galahad, while preparing to unload soldiers, was attacked by 3 A4 Skyhawks from the Argentinian air force. It was set alight, killing 48 soldiers and seamen. Would these parents ever get this chance to visit their sons, resting place again?

It was a poignant time when we sailed passed the islands that day. It was also Remembrance Sunday, November 9th. The weather brightened and calmed a little in the late afternoon so a memorial service was held at sea on deck. It was very emotional, as one can imagine, and Dave and I, along with other passengers near the rails, were given a small wooden cross with a poppy on and asked to throw them overboard, after the Captain and other dignitaries had thrown memorial wreaths overboard. When the time came we all duly did as asked except for Dave who just couldn't let go. We waited until the service was over and all the passengers and crew had dispersed and then, knowing we were alone, he was able to throw it overboard saying his own prayer.

One of the highlights of the cruise was sailing into Rio Di Janeiro and the sight of the sun shining on Sugar Loaf Mountain. We were in carnival country and Dave's love of music and dancing was increasing so where better to practise.

There were no carnivals on while we were in port, but they have a carnival school and theatre so that's where we went that evening. The music was a loud samba beat, intoxicating in itself and the colours of the costumes were so vibrant. When the girls sashayed down the stage steps looking for volunteers to teach how to samba, guess who was one of the first up needing no persuasion? Yes, it was Dave. I found this lack of inhibition hard to cope with in the early days as he used to be a little quiet with strangers and certainly not what you would call a ladies' man. It took a while to realise that being outgoing and larger than life was normal behaviour for a lot of people, including myself at times, and I was going to have to get used to this new Dave. He was certainly most enthusiastic about learning to samba with this gorgeous scantily clad six foot two Brazilian lady. His enthusiasm didn't reach his feet though as I felt sure he was going to trip both of them up at one point. 'Best night of my life', he said on the way back to the ship. This was to become a regular saying of his; best meal, best day out, best holiday, best party etc. Such was his love of life and Alzheimer's could just wait.

Before we left Rio we visited Ipanima and I've never heard so many people hum that song, The girl from Ipanima in one day. Walking along the beach Dave decided he needed a haircut. So, walking up a backstreet, we found a hairdressers with a very attractive young lady inside. She was the receptionist so when a short, chubby, young lady with frizzy hair appeared Dave grinned at me in the mirror. Sure enough when we got home he was describing her exactly like the girl in the Samba theatre. 'The most gorgeous Brazilian girl cut my hair', he would say. He loved the thought of being in exotic Brazil so he had to tell friends how beautiful his Brazilian hairdresser was.

Towards the very end of this amazing voyage while cruising the Atlantic towards home we took part in a celebration of 'The renewal of marriage vows' along with four other couples.

The most poignant part being 'in sickness and in health' and you know, although it was an emotional service, we didn't feel sad at that vow, but quite the opposite and very positive. We had just had the most wonderful holiday, something we would never have dreamed of.

The two of us on the QE2. Who would have thought it?

Chapter 13

ACCESSING CHARITIES

As time went on, although Dave continued his determined efforts to keep up his skills, It was a struggle when he had forgotten to do something as simple as make a cup of coffee. If he did remember he would repeat the procedure and would make as many as 3 cups which I would find in various parts of the kitchen.

If I went out with friends for a couple of hours I would put soup or stew in the microwave with the timer set and a green sticker on the start button. This worked for a while, and then I had to leave a sandwich. Other carers had told me if they left anything their partners often forgot to eat but that's one thing Dave never forgot to do.

His inability to do certain things frustrated him and often caused him to lose his temper. I accessed a charity called PPS in Liverpool which provides aids to independent living. We got a photo phone (small frames on the phone showed a photo of the person he wanted to speak to) so he simply had to press a button. There was also a speaking clock, but he often couldn't locate the buttons on these things. He also had a speaking watch on which he could locate the button.

He would press the button at the most inappropriate time; once in the theatre, several times in the cinema and sometimes while having a meal out. The voice recording was tinny with an obscure accent and people would turn around to see where it was coming from. So I learnt to look around, as if as puzzled as they were.

Needing the toilet when we were out was a problem as I needed to help Dave. Having a radar key was helpful and also meant there was plenty of room. If there was no disabled toilet I quickly learned that the only way was to walk straight into the ladies ,explain the situation briefly and use their disabled toilet .We would find a way of overcoming any problem rather than stay at home.

Although I was having some respite, as Dave worsened I needed more help. One day after a particularly difficult morning, I was in St Helens walking passed the MIND office. I didn't know an awful lot about this mental health charity but I called in to see if they could help me. I was desperate. Only that morning Dave had become incandescent with rage and had refused his daily medication. I pleaded with him to take a diazepam tablet, which was to be given only when things got out of hand. Glass of orange in hand, tablet in the other I was trying to persuade him that he would feel so much better if he took it.

'NO', he roared, lashing out at me.

So without another thought I popped it into my mouth and washed it down with the orange. One of us was going to feel better!

Within a short time of talking with a young lady on reception I was feeling much better. She wasn't just concerned about Dave; she wanted to talk about me, because of course, caring can affect one's own mental health and wellbeing.

Realising that the time had come when I could no longer leave Dave for any length of time, suggestions for relaxing therapies for me were limited unless I accessed more care. We talked about the benefit of exercise and how it would release endorphins making me feel less stressed. That was something I should have been doing anyway as I attended the rheumatology clinic where my physiotherapist was always telling me the importance of finding time to do the exercises she set for me. My nurse practitioner also, knowing my situation with Dave, at each appointment would spend some time talking of the importance of learning to be kind to myself.

This is something most carers have a problem with. As this dreadful disease develops, the workload gets heavier; there is lack of sleep, irritability and subsequent guilt. I realised that it was time to access more care and, although Alzheimer's was not something MIND had dealt with before, they were prepared to help.

Walking into the MIND office that day was the best thing I did throughout Dave's Illness and the timing couldn't have been better as they were preparing to open a council owned allotment. Dave could get involved with gardening again.

The first couple of times he went his brother Derek went with him. Volunteers were in the process of erecting a huge polytunnel in absolutely foul weather. Having met some of the volunteers in the office Dave was quite happy to have me drop him off for a couple of hours and pick him up later. There was always a cup of coffee on offer in the shed and when the warmer weather came it was relaxing sitting in the sun with no rush to go home as Dave was always happier in company.

One of the memories we can laugh about, is when there was a mound of top soil to be sifted and moved and Dave took spades of it further and further away, putting it goodness knows where. One of the founder members of Mind in St Helens became manager of the allotment, dealing with any council issues or developments. MIND are now the proud owners of a new shed and their own toilet. Martin is another tireless worker who spent his 80th birthday party on the allotment this year. Dave wore a baseball hat with 'Head Gardener' written on the front and Martin used to tease him saying he should be wearing it, but Dave wasn't having any of that.

There is now a brass plaque on a picnic bench at the allotment. It reads 'IN MEMORY OF DAVE CRANK (HEAD GARDENER) ALWAYS MADE OUR DAYS HAPPIER.' When at a trustees' meeting I was told of the plan I shed a few tears. What a wonderful thing to do in his memory.

One of the volunteers, Dene, became Dave's new best friend and a major part of his life. She is the hardest working volunteer I know and as well as being involved with the allotment runs a ladies' craft group, trips out on a barge, social evenings and helps them save for a holiday each year which she books and organises. Often when it was almost time to go and collect Dave she would ring and say, 'I'm just going to (wherever). Is it o.k. to take Dave?'. So I would get another couple of hours and maybe she would stay for tea. This was all so important for Dave as the more social interaction he had the better.

There was also a men's group organised by MIND on a Monday morning. Two of Mind's activity workers would facilitate the group having quizzes, football discussions, a film or Dave's favourite card game, chase the ace. Prompted by a volunteer, if he won the £1 he was delighted. As a result of Dave's involvement I am now a trustee with MIND, and although when in meetings I am constantly having to ask Jean the office manager, or Bernard the Chairman, to explain certain things, one thing I have learnt is that according to anecdotal evidence there has been a massive decrease in hospital admissions for people with mental health problems who have accessed MIND.

At Dave's funeral a man approached me saying, 'Dave was so good to me on the allotment; he became my friend'.

I was told this man had been on a train for the first time in his life the week before with one of the volunteers who befriended him. It was amazing that as Dave was approaching the late stage of Alzheimer's he was able to befriend someone and make them feel good about themselves.

From MIND I was advised to go to ST.HELEN'S CARERS CENTRE, another charity that became a lifeline. They offered carers a number of courses. The first course I did there was a basic computer course but then I concentrated on the other training courses on offer. I did the YESTERDAY, TODAY, TOMORROW certificate, the SUPPORTING THE DEMENTIA JOURNEY course and the ALZHEIMER'S CERTIFICATE. All of these courses had many 'penny dropping' or what I call 'light bulb' moments. When certain situations were illustrated I could understand why things became confrontational. I am only human and even with training the unexpected incident could still stress me out.

It wasn't just the training courses that helped but the social side of the Carers Centre with the fortnightly dementia support group where one of the staff Joanne became like a friend. Always ready to help with a smile she resolved many issues. A Garden party in a marquee in the summer, an hilarious pantomime at Christmas, relaxing therapies, and days out during carer's week. These treats or days out were taken for granted before dealing with Alzheimer's but had now become something to really look forward to.

We also had support from another group now called 'MAKING SENSE', which was originally an

Alzheimer's support group which had transferred to the town centre. There was a demand to keep it open and it relaunched under a new name. Organised by experienced trained professionals in dementia care, we would meet on the second Tuesday of every month with or without our partners. Often there would be an informative talk, a meditative therapy or a social evening. Whatever it was, it was always interesting to watch Dave's reaction. He would nod in agreement with a speaker often saying, 'You are so right', even if he hadn't a clue what was being talked about. God forbid if I tried to shush him but often a speaker would engage him in a talk. Dave was always good at bluffing almost to the end.

There is apparently a theory that support groups should meet in an informal setting away from the hospitals and without professional involvement, yet here we were in a hospital environment with four professionals highly trained in dementia care and thriving as a support group with advice on hand at any given time.

One of the nurses, as well as remaining involved with the 'Making Sense' group, is Nurse Specialist In the Care Of Older Persons at another nearby hospital. She and a colleague had developed an initiative called the 'Forget-Me-Not' scheme. The idea was that when a patient was admitted on to the ward a card with an illustration of a forget-me-not flower was placed on the bed frame where it could easily be seen by staff. This card would display information regarding the patient's dietary requirements, likes, dislikes etc.

At meal times patients with dementia would have their meals served on a red tray, thereby indicating that the patient might need help or that the tray was not to be removed until the meal had been eaten. It was a common complaint in the past that trays had been taken away from patients who either couldn't reach them or weren't aware they were there.

Dave having to go into hospital and being frightened in a strange environment was something I tried not to think about, so it was heartening to know there were going to be changes. I once asked the Nurse Specialist if it didn't make her feel despondent when reading negative press reports regarding patient care. 'You just have to keep chipping away at it', she said.

This new initiative was to be launched at the hospital with a party to celebrate it and Dave and I were invited. Once again I think Dave thought this party had been thrown for him as he was warmly greeted by those who organised 'Making Sense'. A cake decorated with forget-me-not flowers was at the centre of the buffet and the room decorated with blue and yellow balloons.

Porters brought patients down from the wards in wheelchairs and a local singer Sandra had been hired for the afternoon. Of course Dave recognised her and presumed, as an old friend, she wouldn't mind sharing the microphone with him. He really needed watching that day as he tried to persuade patients to get out of their wheelchairs and dance.

Senior nursing staff and dignitaries who had attended in an official capacity were also fair game for a dance and Dave wouldn't take no for an answer. It was a brilliant afternoon and as we drove home in the rain I thought how having one of these parties once a week would be so beneficial. We loved it when we were invited to any function, and it was a known fact that we would go to the opening of an envelope.

The Alzheimer's group in its new venue at United Reform Church in St Helens continued to thrive. Managed by Denise and assisted by volunteers they came up with the idea of a sort of breakfast start to the day serving toast and crumpets. Then there might be a quiz, musical bingo or a sing-along. Volunteers interacted with clients using some extra large games like skittles, connect four and curling, while carers had a chat and a cuppa. Some people loved it when we played dance music, especially Dave, even though he bumped into people who took their dancing seriously. Dave enjoyed specialised play equipment e.g. large connect four, skittles and dominoes.

One of the most memorable mornings was Laura's sing-along with an Elvis theme .She had printed the words to all the songs, and believe me there was movement with music and plenty of gyrating. The funny thing was that we hadn't realised that there were schoolchildren in the room above having a fire service talk. A teacher came down to ask if we could we keep the noise down as the fireman's talk couldn't be heard. Imagine the expression on her face on being told that it was an Alzheimer's group being over- enthusiastic.

How glad Dave was that it was music he recognised from an era well remembered. We are moving with the times, though there are many occasions when gentle, quiet, relaxing music is more appropriate.

Without these charities I don't know how I would have coped; they were the reason I was able to keep Dave at home for 10 years and I can't thank them enough.

According to Dementia UK we now have more Admiral Nurses in the North West but they are still only in Manchester, Preston and Knowsley. There are many more employed all over the South. Admiral Nurses support people with dementia and their carers, providing the carer with emotional and psychological support and guidance in accessing services. They also promote positive approaches to living with dementia.

I was fortunate enough to be able to access charities, but imagine being housebound and having to cope with dementia. A visit on a regular basis from an Admiral Nurse would have made so much difference. Why are there so few in the north and so many in the South ?

I have received so much support from Dave's Community Psychiatric Nurse , Jeanette. I once told her she was down on my calendar as one of Dave's activities because her fortnightly visits were so looked forward to. Once again there were no inhibitions on Dave's part as he made it so obvious he adored her from when she first started coming to us. After making sure I knew she was aware of boundaries it was decided to limit Dave to a peck on the cheek on arrival and on departure.

This didn't stop him trying for another one in-between but usually he would try for that when I went to put the kettle on. ALZHEIMERS ??? Or was he just being a red blooded male?

Chapter 14

BECOMING PROACTIVE

We were invited to attend THE ALZHEIMERS SOCIETY CONFEFENCE in Newcastle .We were booked into a hotel, with two other couples from the Southport branch of the Alzheimer's Society. Having booked into the hotel we managed to locate Doris and Harry, who has since sadly died, but didn't meet up with Sue and Richard until the following morning when we were due to leave for the venue.

Walking along crocodile style somebody shouted out, 'Are we all here?' and Richard shouted back, 'Well I'm not'. I realised straight away that Alzheimer's so far hadn't interfered with Richards's sense of humour and he and Sue were to become our great friends.

On arrival at the venue we met even more people coping with the same condition. Each table appointed a scribe and we took notes and shared ideas. I remember thinking it was alright to laugh with someone, who while speaking on the microphone, forgot what he had started talking about. I don't know whether it was this that gave Dave the incentive but he raised his hand to speak when someone was taking the roving microphone around during an open forum. Now at this stage I was nervous when Dave stood up to speak in front of about 400 people. He really struggled and I don't know how much was understood but I know the gist of it was about how important it was to keep trying and not be embarrassed about struggling to speak. He did hesitate a lot and finally dried up and had to stop. Having stopped he was given a resounding round of applause .

When we had a lunch break shortly after several people came up and gave him a pat on the back saying, 'Well done'.

One lady said to me, 'I bet you felt like getting him by the seat of his pants and making him sit down'.

'Not at all', I said. I can honestly say apart from feeling nervous for him when he raised his hand to speak, it was one of the proudest moments of my life.

We had a great day and when we got back to our hotel after dinner we enjoyed meeting people from Scotland and Wales who had been at the conference and even laughed and joked as we tried to guess which partner had Alzheimer's.

That same year we had another great adventure by going on a protest march when there was a threat that NICE would put a stop to the prescribing of Aricept and Memantine, claiming they were not cost effective. Dave and I joined the Southport group on the train at Wigan and there was a happy atmosphere as we all received our leaflets with various protest chants for us to learn.

Arriving at the park in Manchester we congregated with members of various groups of members of the Alzheimer's Society from all over the North. Marshals and officials distributed placards with a variety of protest messages on such as, 'IT'S NOT A 'NICE' DECISION', 'MEMORIES ARE PRICELESS', 'KEEP ALZHEIMER'S DRUGS ON THE NHS'. Dave's placard said, 'AM I WORTH £2.50 PER DAY?'. Oh yes you were Dave, you were priceless.

Before the march started Richard was interviewed for local television and the whole thing was becoming very exciting and, more importantly, there was a feeling we were actually doing something as we literally made our voices heard as we began our slogan chanting. Marshals grouped us together and we began our slow march, chanting and wearing our bright yellow tabards and sashes, through Manchester with a Police escort. Dave was making his own chant up. The whole atmosphere was making Dave a little over excited and I'm afraid occasionally someone got a light knock on the head from his placard so I persuaded him to march on the outside of the group.

We marched along, a policeman at the side of us, and as we slowed down on a corner there was a group of youths who found the sight of us old fogeys hilarious.

'What are you marching for mister?' one of them shouted to Dave.

'DRUGS!' shouted Dave quick as a flash. I didn't have time to register the expressions on their faces as we marched on but the policeman had a broad smile on his face. I guess we were one of the easiest protest marches he had been involved in.

On arrival at the public square there were several speeches regarding the threat to our drugs. We had made our voices heard, the protest was over and thank God they are still being prescribed on the NHS. These drugs gave Dave and me almost ten years of extra time.

Time to enjoy our family, watching our grandchildren grow and leaving them precious memories of their granddad. It meant we could continue for longer enjoying our travels and spending time with friends. Also 10 years of making new friends as we developed our amazing support network.

As the crowd dispersed there was a bit of an anti-climax but this was soon rectified as the Manchester Christmas market was on. So we spent the rest of the day savouring the atmosphere and the food, as we wandered around enjoying the sights, sounds and smells of Christmas.

Having completed my courses at the Carers Centre there was to be a presentation of certificates not just for carers but for various students who had done courses through the local Technical College or Social Services. Another carer and I had been asked to say a few words regarding being a carer. As Dave was my guest at this event I had to choose my words carefully and of course discuss with him first what I was going to say. He was all for it, but it was agreed I would talk about a couple of the more amusing but frustrating incidents that had happened.

He sat on the front row and thoroughly enjoyed the proceedings. Any sign of laughter and he almost stood up and took a bow. When Jane and I were presented with flowers he walked forward giving us a standing ovation. This was the start of a change in Dave's personality where he enjoyed being at the forefront and involved.

Dave's consultant thought it might be an idea if, on one of her study days, Dave and I talked to some students about living with Alzheimer's; the idea being that the students could speak to Dave first and then to me while asking questions about living with dementia, having holidays etc. Dave spoke a little first with some prompting and quite enjoyed the experience. Then his Consultant suggested Dave might like to go for a cup of coffee with a young lady who was sitting at the back of the room.

'No thanks', he said, 'I would rather stay and listen to Joan'. So I was obviously limited in what I could talk about. He obviously knew I would be talking about him as it wasn't like Dave to pass up the chance to go for a coffee with an attractive young lady.

We were then asked by a Nurse Specialist for Older People to take part in a filmed interview for 'The Forget-Me-Not' Initiative. There were several people involved, a Consultant, nurses, voluntary workers and a student nurse all filmed in their working environment, but Dave and I did our filmed interview in our own home.

This film was to be used for training purposes in the Carers Centre and in Care Homes. Dave talked about how on the day he was told he had dementia he died inside, something I had never heard him say before, but then he proceeded to say, 'But you can't die we had the kids'. By this he meant the grandchildren.

I prompted him by asking what we did when feeling low, to which he replied by advocating the merits of Knowsley Safari Park. 'Look at those monkeys and they would make anyone happy', he said. It would have made a good advert for the Safari Park.

There was some confusion as he claimed to have actually flown the helicopter over the Grand Canyon when on holiday, but then he laughed at himself and said, 'But I couldn't have, couldn't I?. He then said something about somebody and I couldn't quite get what he meant.

'Who's that Dave?' I asked.

He leaned back to look at me in disbelief. 'Well you should know', he said.

It was only on viewing this film again recently I realised how this kind of answer was used when he lost his train of thought so I learnt to give an answer like, 'Oh of course, I think I know what you mean'. Meaningful conversation had become a thing of the past and it had happened without me realising it.

In 2010 we were invited to attend a Dementia Care Conference at a hotel. A talk was given by an actress about her personal experience and involvement with her grandmother who had died with dementia. There was also a very charismatic speech from Dr. David Sheard who is Chief executive and Founder of DEMENTIA CARE MATTERS. He is also an advocate of positive personal dementia care and has written several books in the 'Feelings matter most' series. After listening to his presentation I realised why he has the reputation as a charismatic speaker and he certainly held Dave's attention.

The filmed interview we had been involved with was shown on a large screen and I don't think Dave could quite believe it. The credits rolled to the accompaniment of 'Always Look on The Bright Side Of Life', and a huge round of applause. We all agreed that Dave had stolen the show that day. The speakers asked to be introduced to him and, as it had been pointed out that we were sitting at the front, he was photographed and several people who were there had been on Dr. Frances's study day. Dave was being treated and behaving like a celebrity and I felt so proud of him that day.

Some mornings he woke up in such a muddle and everything was an effort, yet he never stayed in a low mood for long and here he was enjoying helping professionals see a little of what life with dementia is like.

Chapter 15

CANADA AND ALASKA 2004

We did try just one more long haul flight to realise two more of our retirement dreams before it was too late. We regarded ourselves as members of THE SKI CLUB (Spending the Kids Inheritance) and it was with their blessing that we continued to do just that as long as we were safe. So what were the dreams? Canada and Alaska where we visited the cities of Montreal, Quebec, Ottawa and Toronto. Seeing Niagara Falls, where we sailed precariously on the Maid Of The Mist, bobbing up and down like corkscrews in the rain wearing the obligatory bright blue plastic mac. From there we flew to Banff where Dave was so excited to be touring The Rockies.

Arriving in Calgary we were met at the airport and transferred to our hotel but en route we would make a stop at a Heliport where those who had booked a flight over the Rockies would leave the coach and the rest of us continue the journey to our hotel, where we would check in and have a look around Calgary.

Dave and I had discussed whether or not to do a Rockies flight when booking the holiday and I had (or thought I had) persuaded Dave that it would be too much for us being in such close proximity with strangers and, being honest with him, I told him I felt that struggling to strap him in was an unnecessary stress for me. We both agreed, until the bus stopped to let those who had booked for the flight to get off and Dave stood up to experience the flight too. He started to get cross with me when I tried to reason with him and of course he had forgotten all about the discussion we'd had.

Fortunately two young sisters from Yorkshire had come to my aid at an earlier comfort stop, when I needed their assistance to guard the ladies toilet door. For some reason Dave had wanted me to go into the gents, and I thought the ladies would be less embarrassing for me.

They knew our situation and offered to accompany him on the flight if there was a spare seat. There was, and he went, leaving me with my heart in my mouth until he was returned to me where I sat on the hotel wall waiting for him. He was so excited about the whole experience when he got off the bus, having made friends with the couple who sat opposite him and the girls on the flight. They were Joan and Bob or 'The Geordies' as Dave called them and along with the girls they were to become our holiday buddies. That was a good start early on for me, as the success of our holiday always depended on the people we met and fortunately we usually met nice people.

Unfortunately the same couldn't be said for our driver who, when I explained the situation to him, looked at me with an expression I couldn't read but it certainly wasn't reassuring. I don't think he spoke to Dave for a couple of days and he certainly didn't endear himself to me for a while, yet I watched as he interacted with other passengers in a humorous way .

If I ever did approach him to ask anything of interest he would adopt a very serious manner when talking to me. Once he got used to us he was alright. I think he was afraid and perhaps he hadn't come across dementia before. His attitude didn't spoil anything as we were making more friends every day, unavoidable with Dave's friendly manner and lack of inhibition. To think he used to be quiet and reserved with strangers.

The initiative that David Cameron spoke of, 'Dementia Friends', where with some training from The Alzheimer's Society, volunteers can make the public more aware of dementia, by talking to various groups, will hopefully make a difference.

Alzheimer's now has a high profile in the media and maybe it's the fact that people in the public eye are sharing their experience on t.v. and in books that is making a difference. Whatever it is, it's a positive attitude toward people with any form of dementia and their carers which helps them get the most out of life.

The next day we visited Lake Louise in Banff National park with its beautiful turquoise water and stunning Alpine backdrop. Dave tried to get too near and slid down a muddy slope for a photo. 'Well everyone else is doing it', he said.

Travelling along the spectacular Ice Field Parkway in Jasper, we stopped at the Ice Field for a ride on an ice explorer onto Athabasca Glacier. There we were in the middle of this huge Icefield with pristine white snow and gulleys of what appeared to be running blue water.

Someone from back home had experienced this holiday with a more upmarket company than our budget one. They had been given whisky in crystal glasses and told to help themselves to the running water. Knowing this I thought it would be fun to buy half a bottle of Scotch and some paper cups to share and had come prepared. Dave delighted in handing the cups around and was everyone's best friend that day.

That last night in Victoria was Dave's birthday and we had a get together in the hotel before we went our separate ways. Our lovely friends, the girls from Yorkshire, had bought him a pair of boxer shorts with a picture of a huge fish in the back with 'NICE BASS' printed underneath and everyone made a fuss of him, which he loved.

We said our farewells the following morning before we boarded the Holland America Cruise ship and felt confident that Joan and Bob and several other fellow tourists would be aboard and it didn't take long to seek them out.

Sailing along the Alaska Panhandle and coastal British Columbia we relaxed, enjoying the incredible scenery as the ship took all day gliding through the Inside Passage of Alaska. Our first port of call was Juneau, Alaska's capital, at the foot of grand mountain peaks, which looked so pretty it was like something out of a film set.

We wandered around looking in shops as they were so different to the big shops we were used to, when Dave spotted a sweatshirt with wolves and the word 'ALASKA' embroidered on the front. Going into the shop to try it on my heart sank as I saw how cluttered it was, even the changing room had a mop, bucket and cleaning equipment in it. It had to be tried on for size as it was quite expensive and this is where the frustration began.

I managed, with a struggle, to get his top off and the new one on, but struggling to get it off I suggested he leave it on while I paid for it. But no, he wanted it off and, starting to shout, he kicked the bucket and wouldn't let me help. We finally got it off, I got his other one on and proceeded to pay. At this point he stormed out of the shop shouting, 'I don't want it.

I continued with the transaction as it seemed the easiest thing to do, making a mental note never to enter a shop again on this holiday. When I got out of the shop he was furious so I just walked ahead towards the ship, as he refused to accept reassurance or even my apology for the shop being cluttered and the bucket being there.

We boarded the ship and when we got to the cabin he took the bag containing the sweatshirt and squashed it into the bin, then stormed out of the cabin. I had to follow him hoping the cabin maid wouldn't find it and keep it, thinking we had made a bad choice. I needn't have worried as when we returned she had laid it out on the bed.

After I had a word with the activities coach Dave spent the rest of that afternoon playing deck games while I relaxed. When I went to collect him before dinner he was a different person, hugging and kissing me telling me how great I was and what a brilliant day he'd had. He did wear that sweatshirt though for years to come and he loved it. Can't think why my son-in-law didn't want to inherit it

With Joan and Bob we experienced a railway trip hoping to spot black bears but as it was so misty they couldn't be seen behind the high chain link fence. Dave took great delight in copying Bob as he roared imitating a bear. We did see the cutest little brown baby bear run across the road though and, to Dave's delight, from the coach window a wolf in the wild. One of his best days. At Christmas we received a card with a photo of Dave and I with a cartoon bear looming behind us and speech bubble coming from my mouth saying, 'I bet those Geordies spot a bear before we do'. I wasn't sure if Dave would remember them but he did. 'Best day of my life', he said, once again.

At last we reached the breath-taking sight of Glacier Bay National Park with huge chunks of floating blue ice and enormous peaks. The huge ship turned around ever so slowly, as though it was a car in a cul-de-sac. This was another jaw dropping moment for Dave as he didn't know whether to look at the scenery or follow the manoeuvring of the ship.

To see rivers of ice, like waves frozen in time, was unbelievable. We cruised through the National Park wondering at the sights nature had bestowed. No wonder it had received world heritage status. 'Best day of my life', said Dave as we came to the end of another perfect holiday, despite any problems that had arisen.

Chapter 16

NEW ZEALAND 2006 AND 2007

On one of our visits to Singapore I decided to accept a frequently offered invitation to visit my old friend Marg in New Zealand. 'You're not that far away', she would say to me on one of our phone calls. She made it sound like catching a bus. Always a very persuasive character she got me thinking about it.

Having been a Manager and co-founder of a Care Home in Whangerei, specifically for people with dementia, she had given me lots of food for thought on how to handle confrontational situations. 'It's you who will have to learn how to step into Dave's world', she said. It was through Marg that I first learned of the expression, 'sun downers syndrome'. Evenings were more difficult as Dave became more and more restless. I had been concentrating on keeping him occupied during the day but was now finding evenings difficult.

Apparently in the Care Home Marg worked in they recognised this and regarded females who were restless as waiting for husbands to come home from work or children coming in from school, so they gave them tasks such as peeling potatoes, dusting, generally preparing the lounge or kitchen for homecoming. Men were involved with digging for vegetables or being helped to read a newspaper so that the incessant agitated pacing of corridors was discouraged by distraction.

Having given it some thought, and after talking it over with Dave, I decided that we would make the trip. Little did I know how concerned our daughters were every time I made one of these decisions. It would be great to catch up with Marg. She and husband Keith had emigrated out there with four young sons in 1983, looking for a better quality of life for the boys Keith had thought; Keith had always worked down the pit Sadly he died the year before we went out there.

We spent some time In Whangarei which was surrounded by green hills giving the effect of the town being in a sheltered basin. We had lunch enjoying the local fare and relaxing in the glorious sunshine with Marg's family but not for too long as she had a plan. She had organised a couple of trips out for us starting from Bay Of Islands where we had an apartment reserved for two nights. She drove us there giving us a commentary on the way. Dave was loving every minute of it and I knew the journey from Singapore had been so worth it. We got to the apartment and after a meal decided on an early night as we had a long coach tour the following day. Marg had thought Dave was doing amazingly well and apart from speech difficulties behaving so well. That night on going to bed he patted me on the head but kissed her goodnight.

After breakfast the following day we set off on a coach tour to Tane Mahuta, or God of The Forest, where the oldest known Kauri tree grew. The scenery on the way there was stunning and the walk through the forest magical. The Kauri tree itself was 51 metres high and 14 metres in diameter with an actual staircase carved inside it, which of course Dave had to climb. This proved a little difficult and it then became apparent to our fellow tourists that he had problems, but nothing we couldn't overcome. As usual people were very kind and supportive.

We then headed for Cape Reinga and a ninety mile beach. This beach was renowned for fast turning incoming tides so normal vehicles were prohibited from parking there. There were a few sights of the tops of cars from when people had ignored the warnings and had then to abandon them;   an expensive mistake.

We were quite safe in a purpose-built coach with tractor wheels called the Dune Rider and headed for 'Gum Diggers Park', an area of unusual sporting activities. On the way along the beach the driver stopped the coach and invited anyone who wanted to have a few minutes swim to do so. I immediately got that sinking feeling as I knew Dave would be one of the first to participate and as I am not a strong swimmer, I knew I wouldn't be able to cope.

He already had shorts on so there was no stopping him as he started removing his sandals ignoring my protests. Fortunately one of our fellow travellers assured me he would watch out for him in the huge waves that were rolling in. So off he went and had the time of his life yet again. I often wonder at how many people there are around the world who don't realise exactly how much they contributed to Dave's zest and enthusiasm for life by their willingness to help and share his enthusiasm.

There was even more excitement to come as we approached Cape Reinga's enormous sand dunes. Sand surfing was a sport in this area so, as the boogie boards were being unloaded from the bus, the driver/guide was gathering everyone around for a safety talk. Dave was becoming agitated with me as I was trying to explain the danger without making him feel inadequate. I pleaded with him to wait until I had spoken to the driver and he finally agreed but, as I was asking the driver to intervene, there out of the corner of my eye I spotted Dave almost running up the sand dune, boogie board under his arm. Not once but twice he managed to get away.

Marg was getting photographic evidence and trying not to laugh at the look of horror on my face. He reminded me of the character in the T.V. programme 'Little Britain', except Dave didn't have a wheelchair. While I was trying to explain my predicament Dave had been there, done that and then back by my side wondering what all the fuss was about. Another reason for him to say, 'That was the best day of my life', and another reason for me to say, 'That was the most stressful day of mine', but so worth it.

We had another night at our apartment before exploring a little more of Bay of Islands. Dave chatted to some young Maori people in traditional costume at a museum and then we took a boat trip around the Islands.

Looking in a gift shop he saw a crystal paperweight with a 3D sketch of a Kiwi bird inside it. He immediately wanted to buy it and the fact that it was expensive didn't mean a thing to him as he had lost all sense of proportion when it came to cost.

He began to become aggressive and I could understand his feeling of powerlessness over choice and money so I gave in and bought it. Sometimes it felt like giving in to a badly behaved child, but it went deeper than that. He knew he had worked hard all his life and now he couldn't understand the difference between a penny and a pound and it frustrated him so. I bought the paperweight and as it sits glistening in the sun on my window ledge I am so glad I did. Not that I had a lot of choice when I could see an angry episode about to happen.

Over the years I realised that shopping was something to be done without Dave as he overloaded my trolley with goods I didn't need or he would walk behind me at the checkout carrying something which he claimed was too heavy for me, to the consternation of the girl on the checkout.

On returning back to Marg's home we were greeted by her grandchildren ,who were waiting the return of 'our visitors from England.' Jake had begun to call Dave 'Granddad Dave' and was eagerly waiting for him to climb up the play structure, which could be anything, but that day it was a pirate ship and the two of them would search over the fields with binoculars looking for pirates while the skull and crossbones on the flag fluttered over farmland that became a pirate-ridden sea.

Having experienced so much, we were invited to something completely different. A party to celebrate the launch of a zip wire structure belonging to friends of the family. My main concern was Dave and the zip wire which stretched between two huge trees over a rather muddy pond. However, I needn't have been concerned as he was happy to watch the children and young adults scoot over the pond holding on precariously to the handle. I think the fact that a good run had to be made before taking off dissuaded him as, although he had no sense of danger, he had less energy than in days gone by.

It really was one of those memorable nights as the stars came out in a clear dark blue sky that seemed so vast. 'You really don't know how lucky you are', I thought looking around at everybody, yet they probably did, because I know Marg's family always wanted to share their love of the country they had adopted as their own.

We met Marg's daughter and family before we left and then, on the way back to Auckland airport, she continued to show us wonderful beaches and countryside.

Marg and I were sad when we parted, after all we weren't getting any younger. However, we needn't have been as, intrepid travellers that we were becoming, we were to return a year later to visit the South Island.

Having made it yet again to visit Sue and the family in Singapore, we then went on to New Zealand. After being met by Marg and spending time looking around Auckland with her and her daughter, we then stayed the weekend with another son and his family before flying out to Christchurch to begin our tour of the South Island. Before our flight to Christchurch we all had lunch at a harbour side restaurant, Dave stretched luxuriously in the sun saying, 'I feel like a millionaire with all these yachts around, don't you Joan?'.

Any doubts I had disappeared. Of course I knew there had been some deterioration in Dave's condition, and I'm sure Marg and Jan could see this. I was now having to shower and dress him daily but my reasoning was that if I could do this on a cold winter morning at home I could do it anywhere, as long as we could handle the travelling and social situations. We always discussed this at length and had there ever been any hesitation on Dave's part we wouldn't have continued. Of course going to Singapore to see Sue and the grandchildren had been the biggest incentive.

Having arrived in Christchurch after a relatively short flight without incident, I felt confident but decided not to attend the informal gathering of our fellow tourists as it had been a long day for Dave and an early night seemed a better option.

The following day we made our way to the dining room only to be met by a 'jobsworth' maître de who refused to let us have a quiet table in the corner even when the situation was explained. He insisted we sit with the coach party on the allocated table. In retrospect this was probably a good thing as it threw us in at the deep end and let our fellow guests see what our difficulties were, as I had thought explanations could be given as and when needed.

Friends would say, 'You don't need to be explaining, lots of people do odd things'. I was the one waiting for the odd thing to happen and Dave and I had always been open and honest about the situation. We didn't have to wait long for the first odd thing to happen. Having joined a table for eight and introduced ourselves we were coming to the end of an enjoyable breakfast when the man sat next but one to me asked the waiter for wholemeal toast and when that arrived asked for some lime marmalade.

He proceeded to prepare his specially ordered toast cutting it carefully into triangles when Dave reached across and started eating it. The expression on the man's face was incredulous and no amount of muttering to Dave of, 'That's not yours', made any difference. Dave continued to enjoy the toast. I certainly wasn't going to remonstrate with Dave publicly and embarrass him so I did what I thought was best and told the lady sitting next to me that he had Alzheimer's, making sure the lady next to her heard and by mid-morning the whole coach party knew and I could relax.

Having seen the main attractions of Christchurch we travelled across the Canterbury plains into Mackenzie country and Lake Tekapo, with Dave constantly commenting on the wonderful scenery as we went through Mount Cook National Park until Mount Cook itself came into view. We had boarded the bus in a more relaxed manner as we had got to know many of our fellow travellers . I had managed to have a quiet word with the driver regarding Dave, stressing that I didn't anticipate any problems but as a physical disability can often be clearly seen, unlike dementia, I thought it only fair he should know. What a lovely man and how understanding he was. He had helped care for his mother who had Alzheimer's for many years and had total empathy with me.

We arrived in Dunedin, the 'Scottish City', which was also a university city. There was to be a traditional Scottish Haggis ceremony that evening which involved the haggis being carried in on a tray to the accompaniment of the bagpipes and a Robbie Burns poem being recited followed by a sword dance.

After the dance we were asked if anyone wanted to volunteer in the dance. Kilts and tam-o'-shanter hats (including attached ginger wigs) were provided. Guess who was first to volunteer? Yes, it was Dave and he wouldn't be persuaded otherwise. Seeing him with ginger hair looked so funny, in fact seeing him with hair at all (well he did have some) looked funny. The fact that Dave had little coordination didn't matter as the rest of the guests having consumed wine and the traditional Scottish toast of whisky with dinner, didn't dance much better than Dave but they all had a whale of a time and Dave made many new friends that night and went to bed a very happy man.

The following day we decided to explore Dunedin.

Although there were many optional excursions I felt that after so much touring we would be better taking our time and ambling around the city. Big mistake. Dave was tired and irritable after a late night and whereas he would have been more amenable in company, on our own I began to feel the effects of his bad humour. Negotiating to cross the roads was a nightmare, with Dave refusing to hold my hand. He made his way into a shop to demand an ice cream cornet, which I knew from experience would be difficult to eat walking along the road so I tried to persuade him that we could get one on the way back, when we could eat it sitting on a bench. He was furious with me and stormed out of the shop. I hurried after him as several people looked on with amusement.

I could see after a while that I wasn't going to change his mood by looking at the buildings, and he didn't want to go on a harbour cruise, so I suggested that we make our way back to the hotel for lunch and maybe sit in the garden with a cool drink. All to no avail, I was getting nothing but looks of fury from him.

As we got near the hotel the ice cream parlour came into view so I went and bought him the promised cornet, apparently too late as he flung it into the nearest bin. Then came a game of cat and mouse. I would walk so far, with him refusing to follow, but then he would move a little nearer, then stop again when I slowly moved on. No amount of pleading or cajoling made any difference as I slowly approached the hotel.

When we did get to our room, which was bungalow style in the hotel garden he got into a dreadful rage, punching cushions and throwing things around until, exhausted, he curled up on the bed and fell asleep.

I made a coffee and went and sat in the garden by a little waterfall to try and relax but in no time at all I was in floods of tears. Apparently the driver's room was next door to ours and he had heard the commotion and came out to see if I was alright. I was embarrassed at first but as he shared stories of his mother's frustration and rages I realised I would never be alone in feeling like I did. Carers all over the world are struggling as I was and are learning day by day.

In future I would make sure we would always be in company, and that if there was nothing on the itinerary we didn't have to see every inch of the place we were visiting every day.

I was so glad of the drivers support and company that day and when Dave woke up he was over it, whereas I was still a bit shaken.

The next day we a took lovely scenic route to Queenstown, famed for its attractions for the young: Shotover Canyon, Skydive Paradise, and paragliding, etc. Thankfully Dave opted to join our new found friends on a steam cruiser to explore the Milford Sound, where we could leisurely view the delights of this Alpine resort and its awesome waterfalls. All went well until Dave did one of his disappearing acts. Several of us searched different parts of the ship until someone shouted, 'Joan, come here quickly'. There was Dave, having joined a party of Australian Senior Citizens singing Waltzing Mathilda, wearing a bushwhacker's hat, corks and all and really looking the part. He was having a whale of a time. No traumas that day.

All good things come to an end and so we flew back to Singapore for another week with our family, much to the relief of daughter Sue who was glad to see us back in one piece.

I didn't think Sue had seen a great difference in Dave but of course eating out had become a problem. Matthew introduced his granddad to Korean food and the children always helped him choose when eating at the Hawkers centre. They were given a couple of dollars and would each go to the food bar of their choice, but this had become too noisy and crowded for Dave.

Then it was another tearful farewell to Singapore and the family, but not for long as they would soon be coming back to England. So it was home for us to support groups and assessments and filling our days with stimulating things to do.

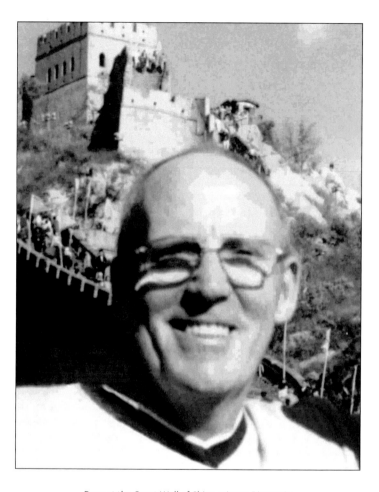

Dave at the Great Wall of China prior to Diagnosis

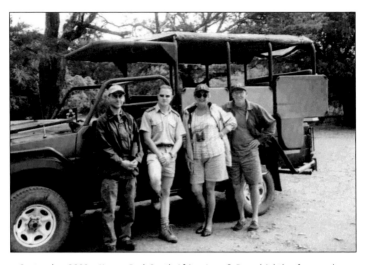

September 2002 – Kruger Park South Africa. Joan & Dave (right), a few weeks prior to diagnosis.

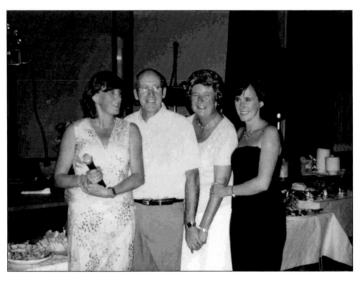

August 2003 – With daughters Jane & Sue, Dave & Joan celebrating their Ruby Wedding Anniversary.

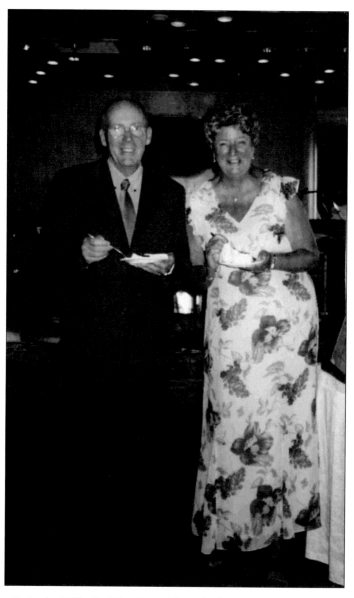

September 2003 – On QE2 eating wedding cake after renewing wedding vows.

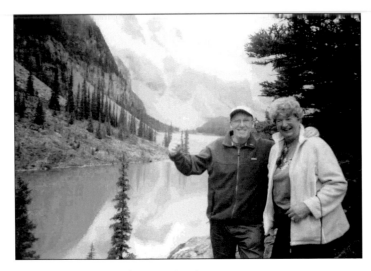

2004 – Dave & Joan at Lake Louise, Canada.

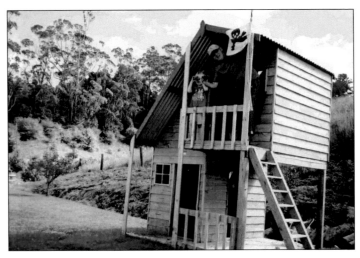

2006 – Dave with his little friend Jake, looking for Pirates in New Zealand.

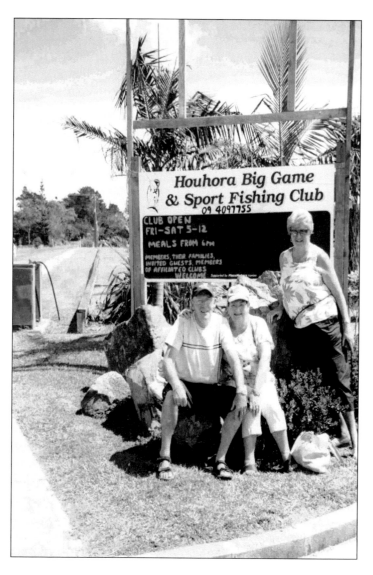

2006 - Taking a break with friend Marg in New Zealand

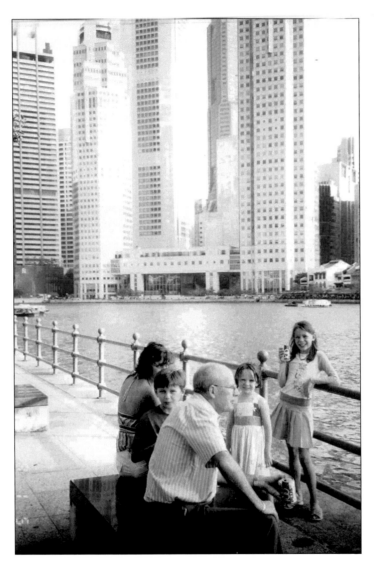

2006 – Singapore visiting family, daughter Sue and grandchildren, Matt, Sophie & Jessica.

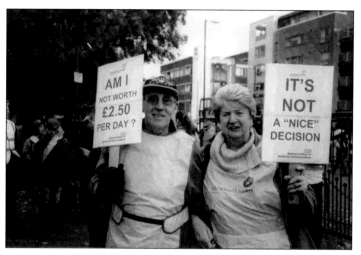

November 2006 – Alzheimer's Society protest march in Newcastle

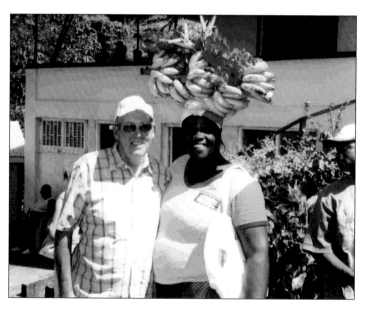

2008 – Cruising The Orinoco Delta and Caribbean

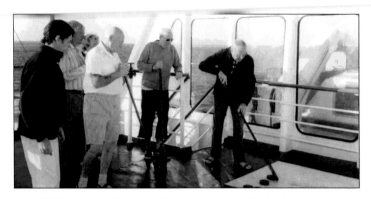

April 2009 – Lands End to John O Groats Cruise on the Black Prince.

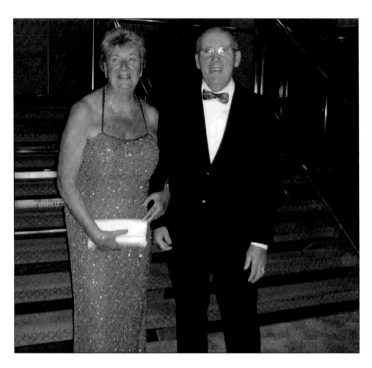

April 2010 – Western Med Cruise.

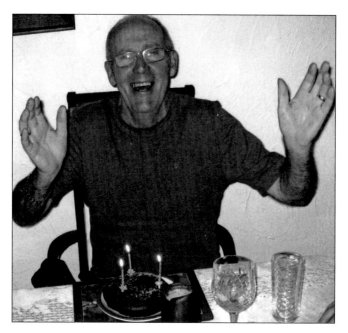

"IT IS I"
August 2011 – Dave's 69th Birthday.

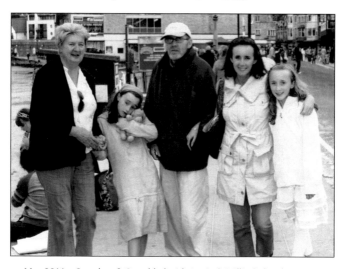

May 2011 – Grandma & Granddad with Annie & Millie & daughter Jane.

Chapter 17

GARDENING AND D.I.Y

We had moved into our house in Billinge in 1965 and regarded ourselves as so lucky to have our lovely new home. Having moved up to Billinge from Liverpool my mum likened it to emigrating, as visiting involved three buses!

With little money and wanting to put our own stamp on the place Dave soon became interested in D.I.Y. and gardening and the garden was soon to become his pride and joy.

Of course, being a newly built house, Dave had to develop DIY skills quickly as money was short, but he was so talented and soon became a man who could turn his hand to anything. Interior decorating was the most difficult though so I would make myself scarce and then, on my return I would casually try to scrutinise the job only for him to shout, 'STOP LOOKING FOR BUBBLES!'

He was just as determined with car maintenance as in the early days we had a succession of old bangers and, with a two bus journey each way to work, a car was a necessity. If he couldn't see what the problem was off he would go to the public library to read a car maintenance book.

The expression in our house from both Sue and Jane if anything got broken was, 'My dad can do anything; he's a fitter'. They had every faith in him, and so did I.

Imagine having been that kind of person, quietly confident, to suddenly in your late fifties start to find life perplexing to say the least. The gardening was the first problem as he repeatedly ran over the lawnmower cable and re connected it. These sort of problems arose within the first two years of being diagnosed. As the cable got more patched up with red tape he blamed the mower and decided that a hover mower would be less problematic. Of course that made no difference, so I persuaded him that a battery operated one would be ideal, always reassuring him that what was happening was no fault of his.

He would get so angry if he couldn't fit the battery properly and I remember Jean next door telling me she had watched him struggling one day until eventually he did let her help. She found it difficult as she knew he was always aware of his limitations.

Of course it wasn't only doing our garden that had become a problem. Dave had, for some time, been doing the garden of our elderly neighbour Frances, who lived in the bungalow opposite, and afterwards enjoyed her homemade scones and a chat. However, she made it clear that even though he was now unable to do the garden, she would still like to see him for tea and scones, so he continued to pop over and when he could no longer go alone I went with him, and so Frances inadvertently became part of our support system.

Eventually I persuaded him we should have a gardener with the excuse that we were getting that bit older and this way would have more time to enjoy life. So along came Brian who still does the garden now.

Thinking that was the end of the gardening problem I didn't bargain for having a garage full of compost but that became an obsession every time we passed Billy and Enid's who, apart from selling everything but the kitchen sink, sold bedding-out plants and compost. We always got more bedding-out plants than we needed and Dave would plant them wherever he felt like, but the bags of compost were building up to ridiculous proportions in the garage.

Dave would beg me to stop the car and Enid's face was a picture as he demanded another bag. It took me a while to realise that he was simply forgetting his earlier purchases but he would never admit to that, and once he threatened to go on his bike and bring a bag back on the crossbar. The bikes had become a problem anyway as he really wasn't safe on the road and was aware of this himself. So I knew collecting the compost on the bike was an empty threat. Eventually the bikes had to be sold, which was another sad loss.

Now and then, as if to prove to me how necessary all this compost was, he would drag several bags out into the garden and proceed to throw spades full of the stuff on the beds up against the fence until it backed up to a slope. I used to think that one day I'd wake up in a valley of compost. It was heart-breaking in the last couple of years as I had to watch him wandering around his beloved garden unsure of what to do. He would break leaves off now and then or snap pieces of twigs and if I didn't empty his pockets before doing a wash load I would find shiny leaves, twigs, apple or pear cores and foil from biscuits when pegging the washing out.

Our daughter recently reminded me of the time when she had planted some bedding-out plants in the borders in her garden and Dave asked her if he could water them. She agreed and with that he jet washed them out of the soil. He apologised, asked if he could he plant them again and then proceeded to plant them all over the lawn.

Dave was determined to continue doing jobs around the house, and I watched from another room one day, realising he was chiselling a hole in the door frame opposite the door handle. The door had been sticking and he thought this would solve the problem. I could tell by the look on his face he realised how futile his work had been when he tried the door to find it was still sticking.

I was never sure what to do in these situations as to say it wouldn't work when he was trying something made him angry, yet to see him realise what he was doing was a waste of time was heart-breaking. He was so aware of his own inadequacies and would often say, 'I'm getting worse Joan'.

There was the time he was using a screwdriver on the top hinge of a door. When asked what he was doing, 'Fixing it', was the answer. That weekend when Sue and the children were visiting the whole door fell against the table trapping Jessica giving her and the rest of us such a fright. He had loosened the top hinge. So slowly I began to get rid of all the tools, but not before he made the most elaborate contraption that would make our kitchen window burglar proof!

We had been burgled recently so Dave made a sort of T bar with a hinge on that could be forced up against the kitchen widow as extra security. The problem was that the window opened outwards, but rather than tell him this I continued to fit it to the window every night until he forgot about it. Having hidden most of the tools I thought I had lessened the chance of any catastrophe, until Ian from next door came up the drive to find Dave on the roof with one leg dangling over, reaching for the ladder which was a few feet away. Ian had to go up on the roof to guide him down. That night we persuaded Dave that Ian desperately needed a new ladder for work so it was moved to next door's garage.

There are so many stories that are funny in retrospect but the funniest one of all, though it wasn't at the time, was when we both got locked in our wet room. The wet room was built at the back of the garage with a door leading in to the kitchen and was originally a shower room. How glad we were, when the time came when I had to see to personal care for Dave a couple of years later, that all that was needed was the removal of the shower cubicle and the sloping floor and drain put in.

When I found I could no longer handle Dave in the bathroom upstairs I was told, by a Social Worker, there was a waiting time of eight months before assessment of the alterations. I mention this because not all Alzheimer's clients are the same and when there is a sudden deterioration there doesn't seem to be a procedure for emergency plans for alterations. Perhaps I didn't push hard enough but bureaucracy can be wearing.

I wasn't prepared for carers coming in to bathe him at this point as he was becoming more aware of his inadequacies and I wasn't going to add to them. Fortunately I had been working full time for many years and we were able to fund the project ourselves from our savings, but I do feel the dignity and self-respect of people should be taken into consideration when it comes to personal care carried out in the home or elsewhere.

Anyway, back to our wet room experience. Dave and I had developed a routine in the morning where, having brought our clothes down the night before and left them in the kitchen, I would put on our towel robes, help him downstairs and before breakfast both of us would shower. I would go first having helped him clean his teeth. I learnt the art of a two minute shower and then, having put my robe back on, would shower Dave. We used to laugh and liken it to a car wash. That was of course if he was in a good mood which he almost always was.

One particular day we were finished but when I came to open the door I heard the handle fall off the other side and the door wouldn't open. 'Don't panic', I said to myself as my heart was going like the clappers. Swathing Dave in towels and sensing his fear I sat him on the chair and reassured him, 'Don't worry, Jean has got a key, I will shout for her'.

So, standing on the toilet seat with my head stuck out of a very small window, I began to shout her name again and again, thinking someone would be walking their dog and would go to the front and get her. Eventually she came back from doing the school run for her daughter and rescued us. Ian opened the door with a pair of pliers. Thank God I was decent.

Looking at the door he said it needed a new handle so warned us both not to shut the door until he got us a new one. We suspected this was caused by one of Dave's final D.I.Y. jobs. We managed to go all day, using the toilet but not closing the door, which meant following Dave every time he wandered into the kitchen. The following morning I made the mistake of entering the wet room first, saying to Dave, 'Don't shut the'......... CLICK! IT HAPPENED AGAIN. The number of people who have said since, 'Didn't you take your mobile in with you?' Hindsight again.

This time I did begin to panic as I suspected that Jean had gone straight out after the school run. Once again reassuring Dave, I told him someone would come soon but not to worry as we had tap water to drink, a toilet and we were nice and warm.

I must have stood on that toilet seat for half an hour shouting, 'HELP! IS THERE ANYBODY THERE? PLEASE COME TO NUMBER 11' .Of course it was bin day and the noise of the lorry and bins drowned my voice out which was going hoarse by now. I don't know what I would have done if the bin man had come up the path as I had no key. In between all this I hit on the idea of a sing-along before Dave started getting agitated. 'Always look on the bright side' was of course a favourite. I was leaning my head on the window frame in despair after another bout of shouting while Dave said the Lord's Prayer, when I heard a gentle voice say, 'Hello, are you shouting for someone?' Was I shouting!

It was our neighbour from the house opposite. Realising our predicament she rang her builder who had been doing some work on her house and he came, gave me some pliers through the window and told me how to release the lock. I opened the front door to return the pliers to a handsome young builder, 'Well I never expected to be rescuing a damsel in distress this morning', he said. No, I thought and I bet you never expected it to be a couple of pensioners neither. Oh the relief when Ian put the new handle on that night!

Chapter 18

SPAIN 2008 AND 2009

Our close friends Pat and Arth had decided to retire and live in Spain and I knew this would have a big effect on our support system, but was grateful that we still had the support of close friends and family. As long haul holidays had become a thing of the past I reassured Dave that we would visit Pat and Arth via one of the budget airlines from the local airport as I knew their leaving was sad for him. There were only three days difference in age between Dave and Arth and apart from spending family holidays together when the children were small they had also shared birthday celebrations. We always made a real do of it if it was a special birthday but my favourite photo is of when they were thirty and Marg, our photographer and friend, took a picture of them cutting the cake as they smiled into the camera. It looked for all the world like a gay wedding.

To visit them I knew I would need support so I was delighted when another one of our circle of friends agreed to come. In fact we managed to go there twice, in 2008 and 2009. Pat had an accident breaking her wrist in 2006 and Dave temporarily became her gardener. Although she had to watch him with the mower cable, he had loved being useful and when her caste was off, it was Pat who bought him his baseball hat with Head Gardener written on the front.

I felt confident about sharing a villa with her and, as it was opposite Pat and Arth's, it would be great. We had a really relaxing time there eating mainly at Pat and Arth's, sometimes at friends of theirs, and a couple of times at their local Chinese restaurant known as 'cheapy Chinese' for obvious reasons. Once, when Dave and Pat were entering the Chinese, Dave let the door go in a man's face and the man was quite angry. When Pat explained about his Alzheimer's the man was mortified. I told her I was often in the position where I didn't know whether to explain or not when incidents like this happened, as I hated making people feel embarrassed.

We have always talked about Dave's awareness of his illness and how upsetting it was. Pat once saw him taking the bin bags to the communal bins at the end of the road. 'This is all I'm fit for now', he said to her with a shrug.

We were all sitting on the beach in glorious Spanish sunshine and Dave turned to me and said, 'See you don't have to go abroad to get weather like this'.

Walking along the water's edge someone asked directions to somewhere and Dave proceeded to give them, pointing up the beach, although he'd never been there before, but Arth took over. Sharing the villa worked out really well and apart from Dave constantly getting rooms mixed up (well she is an attractive blonde and quite a few years younger than me)we had no problems. After a few years they decided to return to

England and I was so glad to have them back in our support system.

I have written a lot about holidays but Dave was always eager to go until his last year and it was something that kept us both going. Friends laughed when I came home and said I didn't think I could do it again as things had been a bit tricky and they always used to say, 'Until the next time'.

Chapter 19

PONTINS 2010

We had a bizarre holiday in 2010 when the Carers Centre asked if we would care to take up the offer of a free apartment with Pontins in Wales at the opening of the season, 'Been there, done that I thought', but when we talked about it we thought we could support one another and it would be a laugh. There were eight of us including one with a mobility scooter and she was a carer. We were four couples all with different problems. One, originally from Trinidad had experienced racial prejudice when he first came to this country 50 years before and as he dipped into his long term memory he was paranoid that staff were not clearing our table because he was black. He also used to be a minister and would often call out, 'Praise the Lord', or 'Alleluia', and sometimes Dave would join in. I remember one particular night when we watched a show put on by the entertainment staff, which was panto style with a lot of audience interaction and frenzied activity on stage. At one point the main character faced the audience wringing his hands shouting 'what shall I do. What shall I do?'

At which point Ricky, in all seriousness bellowed back with his Caribbean accent 'YOU MUST TAKE CONTROL'.

'Be quiet' his wife said.

We were all so used to being on guard in public, and watching out for behaviour problems, that being together seeing the funny side, or the bright side as Dave would call it, was really refreshing. There was also someone there who attended the same day care centre that Dave was attending at the time. He was a retired policeman, but somehow thought he was working at the day-care and was constantly reassuring me that Dave was doing well and that he was doing his best for him. Then there was another one who was constantly demanding his driving license back and becoming more and more confused over whether his mother was alive or not. He was a keen snooker player and he and Dave used to know one another from the local club but his wife and I were never sure whether they remembered that or not .The first night there was a bit chaotic as he kept wandering off to see a football match on T.V. Dave would follow him with me close behind and then one of the others would tell me to go and sit down as he would look after them. Ricky was cold and wouldn't take his hood down which, when the lights went down for the show, was a bit scary as he looked like Darth Vader. All together we looked like a scene from 'One Flew over the Cuckoo's Nest'.

There was a quiz on stage one night and one of the Bluecoats (entertainment staff) was shouting out for names of teams but they had to be called after beans. It was for children really and they were volunteering names like French beans, runner beans etc. 'What about you lot?' one of the Bluecoats shouted to us.   He'd been chatting to us all week and for such a young man had made a real connection with us.

'The has Beans', I shouted, after we'd had a group discussion so that's what we became known as for the rest of the holiday.

We did manage to trundle down to the beach as a group, Marlene on her mobility scooter Ricky on his stick and the rest of us leaning against the wind on a cold blustery day. 'Not like Trinidad here, Is it Ricky, shall we go back?' I said.

'Praise the Lord', said Ricky.

It rained most of the time, and a lot of our spending money went on feeding the meter for heating in the chalets but we did have some laughs. Of course our problems went with us and when Dave had a bout of aggression at the end of one evening, Brenda told me next day that she was prepared to have to come and intervene as she had never heard Dave like that and it frightened her. But the next day Dave was happy as Larry. As anyone who has stayed in a holiday camp knows, the walls are paper thin. We had our main meal together in the restaurant after the busy lunchtime rush was over and it was quiet, so that we weren't concerned how anyone ate and Dave could finger feed to his heart's content. When leaving we said our farewells to the staff, letting the young man in charge of entertainment know what a positive influence they had been. Pontins and St Helens Carers' centre had given us all a memorable Freebie.

Chapter 20

CARDS AND PRESENTS

Dave had never been a hearts and flowers man, or one for booking romantic meals or weekends away, yet that didn't stop me knowing that the love we had for one another was so strong for the almost forty nine years we were married. He didn't believe in Valentine's Day considering it commercialised by card manufacturers, and I thought it ironic when he sometimes brought home a card from respite care that someone helped him make. He had always sent lovely cards at Christmas and on my birthday, and I knew he would be upset at me not getting one when he saw other peoples' cards. So by the year 2003, when he was unable to write or buy a card, I coerced our friend Marj into helping him out. She would make a card on her computer with perhaps a picture of a forthcoming cruise ship or holiday and in the early years of his illness he would tell her the words he wanted on the card. Marj always left me in no doubt that they were his words. She would come to the house with the card and somehow get him to join her in the hall where she would remind him of the occasion. After quite a bit of whispering she would pass him the card and he in turn would turn to me with a beaming smile and say, 'Happy birthday', or 'Happy Christmas Joan'.

Once, he dictated a message on the card to Marj saying, 'I know things have not been very good lately and I want to thank you my Joan for everything you do for me. I love you very much'. The next day he had a major strop, ripped it up and threw it at me. Such is life. I know he meant those words at the time though.

Before his illness he wasn't one for spontaneously arriving home with flowers. If it was a birthday he would sometimes call to Billy and Enid's shop for flowers and I do remember being particularly touched, when just after having to send his driving license back, he went and returned on his bike with a great big awkward looking bunch of gladioli. I can still see that huge grin on his face.

A few years after we first moved to Billinge, Dave had a workmate called Brian who belonged to a horticultural society and grew prize winning Chrysanthemums. Now these are my least favourite flower but every year the time of our anniversary coincided with the time Brian's Chrysanthemums were at their best and he would sell them. Consequently Dave would arrive home with a most untidy looking bunch of flowers wrapped in newspaper and I would smile through gritted teeth as Dave would say, 'But just look at the heads on them Joan, they're enormous'.

As Dave's illness progressed he wasn't able to use the ATM or make a purchase. Presents were easier as we would wander around the shops until I saw something I liked, ask if I could have it and then take him to an ATM to let him see it was his money that was paying for it. So important for his self-esteem.

One gift from him I will always remember for his thoughtfulness. Long before his illness in the 1980's I 'd had a bad year with a back problem and had also developed pleurisy. Having got my size, he bought me a suede sheepskin lined coat with a hood so my back would be warm. We could ill afford it at the time but he got it ,gift wrapped it (with the coat hanger sticking out) and when I opened it I cried. To me that was much more than romantic gesture.

Presents for Christmas were usually sorted out by Sue or Jane and given to Dave to be passed to me, but the last couple of years as he became more confused giving me my present was like playing pass the parcel. The last one Sue passed to Dave, whispering for him to pass it to me. He looked at me, passed it back to Sue who tried again until I got it. All the time he had a smile on his face as if to say, 'I know what I should do but I just don't get it'.   Receiving a gift was only important to me as long as it was important to Dave and he had amazing insight almost to the end.

Although we weren't ones for romantic dinners for two this changed, believe it or not, as Alzheimer's progressed .Sometimes it was easier to stay in and make it special so I would put flowers on the table, light a candle, play some nice music and yes we would even dance after we had eaten. Nothing wrong with a nice smoochy dance. It is said that Alzheimer's steals away the person you love but because Dave had that insight and knew me to the end I never felt I'd lost him altogether. Just that he was different .

Chapter 21

CHANGES IN BEHAVIOUR

As this dreadful disease progressed my ability to stimulate Dave with activities in the home was becoming more difficult. I was grateful for my nursery nursing skills in the early years as setting out work to do after breakfast was second nature to me, but we had now gone beyond jigsaws, colouring in and painting as his dexterity in holding small objects became difficult. He did enjoy it when I read to him for a while, particularly if it was a book about Liverpool in the past, he loved recognising names of roads or areas in Merseyside. I don't think he ever got the story and sometimes I think he just liked the closeness and the sound of my voice.

He also loved, music particularly from the sixties, and I often wonder if the window cleaner caught sight of us having a jive after breakfast. Television was becoming less interesting as he couldn't follow even the soaps. If there was a football match on I would turn his chair to face the T.V. (we had bought a T.V. with a big screen)make him a shandy and put it on a table with a bowl of nuts and crisps. His face would light up and he would settle down to enjoy it, particularly if Liverpool were playing. As soon as the first goal was scored it was all over for Dave. No matter how much I tried to explain that the game hadn't finished he was off to bed. So I would be hoping for a late goal so that he could be occupied and I could keep my nose in my book. The other favourite on T.V was watching a DVD of Les

Miserables. We had seen the show twice years before and he absolutely loved it and became quite emotional watching it.

There were difficulties with visual perception and sometimes he would eat his meal, leaving half of it on the plate and when I turned the plate around he would always look surprised and tuck in once again.

He shaded his eyes in any bright light yet needed the lights on as soon as daylight started to fade. Nor realising at first that it was the damage to the brain that was causing these problems I booked an appointment with his optician who had known Dave from before diagnosis. Testing his eyes was difficult as he couldn't say the letters so Mr Bowen hit on the idea of using pictures. That of course gave him the word finding problem. Though Dave couldn't find the word when looking at the picture of an umbrella, he mimed, wiggling his fingers as though rain was coming down. We were on a roll then and Mr Bowen was so pleased, but Dave didn't need new glasses.

There were difficulties with co-ordination, sitting down on a chair, getting into his seat in the car etc. Sometimes he would get in and then get out and turn around up to three times before I could fasten his belt. I just had to be patient but sometimes he would lose it and say, 'I'm not going'. Other times he would see the funny side of it saying, 'What am I doing?'

On holiday with the MIND group in Cornwall getting him on the coach was so difficult. He had three steps to get up and then we were on the front seat, but he insisted on sitting on the top step, or on the gearstick (he soon got up from that). Once tried to sit on the driver's knee. 'Are you driving then Dave?' the driver said. This was as puzzling to Dave to those around him but sometimes it would cause him to rage.

There had been mood swings and bouts of anger within a couple of years of diagnosis but particularly in the last four years or so the rages and aggressive outbursts were becoming more frequent, giving cause for concern to all who cared for and supported us both.

In the early years I often reflected and blamed myself for an outburst as I wouldn't consider patience and tolerance to be my finest qualities, but after a while I do think what was my weakness became my strength. I had to learn patience and tolerance for both our sakes and to realise that Dave needed constant reassurance. He also needed to know how much he was loved by everyone and that we still had plans for days out or even holidays.

Of course caring takes its toll and there were times when I woke up in the morning thinking that I didn't want to get up and do the bathing /showering routine, particularly if I had been up a couple of times during the night with Dave. Then I would hear the shout from the other room, 'Is there anybody in this house?' and I would go in to find a smiling Dave, but sometimes it would be a look of fear or anger. At times like this I was having attacks of anxiety. I had been prescribed beta blockers for the first time in 2004, to be taken as and when I felt the need, which was until Dave died and for a while after. The following year I was diagnosed with Hypertension, having never had blood pressure problems before. Most of the carers I know are on some form of medication as this cruel illness takes its toll on the carer and the cared for.

There was always a fear of him falling downstairs so we got a pressure mat, which whenever he got out of bed set an alarm off in my room and also shone a white light which often woke me up before the alarm sounded.

I had moved into another room in 2007 because Dave was so easily disturbed, but also because with his illness he had developed twitching and jerking movements that kept me awake. If ever he got distressed then I would get in his bed to cuddle his back and we would both drift off, only for him to do one of his jerks and frighten the life out of both of us. So back I would go to my own bed. I used to joke that it was like playing musical beds, playing down the fact that I had lost another part of our marriage. The love was still there, but during the night if he became frightened I had to give him all the emotional support while I felt such turmoil inside.

If he was in a bad mood in the morning he would resist my efforts to get his clothes, on yet would complain of the cold and be unable to help himself. On days like this I would cover him in the duvet and bring breakfast up on a tray so that hunger wouldn't make him worse. When I came into the room with the tray I would have my, 'let's start again', smile on and sit down chatting and more often than not he would say, 'Well this is nice'.

Yes, there were times when I feared for my own safety. It was o.k. for him to kick doors and walls, but if it escalated and showed no sign of abating then I would ring for help. Jean next door was my first port of call but if it was in the evening I would ring his brother or sister as they were often due to come anyway. Of course I never told Dave I had rung, so it would look as if they had turned up spontaneously, but although it took no longer than twenty minutes to half an hour for them to arrive Dave would still be in a state of distress.

Discussing this with them recently, sister in law, Ella said she remembered one particular time when Dave just kept repeating, 'I'm sorry, so sorry', while breaking his heart crying on his brother Derek's shoulder. I was sitting on another chair crying bitterly, exhausted and at the end of my tether. Ella said, 'You have absolutely nothing to be sorry for Dave'. His insight was such that when the rage was over he was mortified at his own behaviour, and my own self-doubt was such that I would wonder how it had got to this and if I could have handled it better. His sister Barbara remembers arriving when I was attempting to give him a diazepam. He wouldn't take it for me but he took it for Barbara. Usually when incidents like this occurred as he calmed down and natural conversation took place, always including him, he would relax and apologise again as they were leaving. When they had gone he would start apologising to me, telling me how much he loved me. I always made sure he understood that he couldn't help it and that it was this horrendous illness that did this. The effect on both of us was devastating but we always bounced back.

One particular time, he was careering around the house in such a rage   I was desperate to get away, so I told him I was going to friends in the next road for a coffee but would come back soon. I wasn't there long when Marj came to tell me she'd had a phone call from a neighbour and that Dave was walking up the road shouting, 'JOAN, JOAN!' at the top of his voice causing the neighbours to be concerned. Marj and Marie persuaded me to stay and finish my coffee while they reassured him. I couldn't settle so drove back round to find a house full. Ciara from next door, Chris from opposite plus friends Pat, Marj and Maria were all doing their best to calm him down, but he was overwhelmed and I persuaded them, with Dave's reassurance, that they could go and all would be well.

Not so. A few minutes after they left he was furious again kicking doors, punching walls, so I rang Pat and once again she and Maria came round in the car. When he saw the car come up the drive he was livid. Ringing for help again was a hard decision to make, as in retrospect, I knew he had been overwhelmed by the friends and neighbours in the house just a few minutes earlier. We needed calm but I was incapable of getting it and he was going out of control again. As Pat and Maria arrived Dave suddenly started stripping off. Already barefoot, off came the sweater and t shirt, and as our friends entered the lounge, down came the trousers, boxers and all. While doing this he kept repeating, 'I haven't got a pin, not a pin'.

I'm not a psychologist but I strongly felt that I could interpret what he meant. In the early days when he kept losing his money and debit card we agreed that he shouldn't have a debit card as, apart from the fear of losing it, he was writing his pin number down on pieces of paper and leaving them in pockets or his wallet. The amount of money he carried had to be reduced as he would lose notes. This was done tactfully as he realised he couldn't help doing this and, as we were always together anyway, I would pay, always assuring him it was from his savings, but I know he found this hard to accept.

When he was sad, angry, or just feeling sorry for himself, and God knows he had reason to be, he would say to me or anyone who cared to listen, 'I haven't even got a pin', and empty his pockets. I would always try to give him some coins but he would say, 'That's slummy', (slang for loose change). Somebody once suggested I give him some foreign currency but his insight was such that I couldn't risk it as it would have been the final insult, to patronise him like that. So what did, 'I haven't got a pin', mean?

In the early days I don't know whether it meant money, or his pin number to get money or even 'penny to my name', which he also sometimes said. What I strongly feel is that on the awful night when he went out of control and began to strip off it was almost like he was saying 'Here, have the lot I've got nothing, not even a pin (or a penny)'. It was devastating, the futility of it all. Even writing about it now chokes me with emotion. Of course my priority was to get him upstairs where he immediately got under the duvet. Having somehow calmed him down and persuaded him to take a diazepam he began to drift off through exhaustion before his medication took effect.

Having finally got downstairs to my friends one of them made a cup of coffee and we began to mull over the events. As always they were voicing their concerns, and as always I was trying to reassure them that everything would be alright the following day. Dave's dignity had been preserved. I had got him upstairs and Pat and Maria had gone into the lounge before he got completely naked but to do this Maria, who was behind Pat, had covered her eyes and in blind panic was bumping into the furniture before I closed the door on them. I can close my eyes now and conjure up the image of Maria stumbling around with her hands over her eyes and it makes me want to giggle.

The following morning I went into Dave to see him peering over the duvet. 'Is everything alright , what happened?', he said. Unlike in any marriage where a bad row may result in the sulks the following day this can't happen with Alzheimer's as the person needs reassurance that it's a new day and everything is going to be fine. Even if I felt resentful I had to fake it to make sure I didn't show it, and that usually worked. As Dave used to say, 'Once we're in the Safari park looking at the monkeys we'll be alright'. And he was right.

Not all changes in behaviour were negative as, although his frustration as his abilities dwindled made him angry and resentful, he remained as friendly and loving as ever when greeting people. So it was even more important that we kept putting ourselves out there in a world which was becoming more and more mysterious to him. As long as it was something I felt he could cope with. So visiting friends and having friends visit was easier than going to restaurants and shows etc. The last two or three years of his illness he still appeared to recognise people but if it was someone involved with his treatment they were greeted as more of an old friend. Our GP had been involved with Dave's care since he finished work after his accident, and had begun to suspect it was Alzheimer's even before the brain scan confirmed it. A visit to the doctor was now like a social occasion and on entering the surgery he would greet her with, 'Hello love and how are you doing'. Political correctness didn't figure in Dave's life. He would then proceed to talk about the latest holiday not forgetting to ask, 'How are you doing anyway love?' Waiting to go into the surgery was a hilarious, especially at Flu jab time, as there would be so many familiar faces I couldn't keep him in his seat as he greeted everyone.

When Dave stopped doing the mini mental health test as his score was so low and it was creating nothing but stress, his Consultant began home visits which Dave loved.

I particularly remember one visit when after enjoying a chat with her she waved as she was getting into her car, and he called out, 'I love you'. On closing the door he said, 'She's a lovely girl you know'. Calling everyone 'love' was a crafty way of not having to think of names but on meeting the Mayor it tickled me when Dave called him mate. This familiarity and friendliness of Dave's helped when I decided to chance going on another cruise and it worked out well as we made friends so easily that we continued to cruise for quite some time.

Chapter 22

THE CRUISING YEARS BETWEEN 2004 AND 2010

It had been quite some time since we had done the South American cruise on the QE2 but I reasoned that although touring holidays like those we had done in New Zealand and Canada/Alaska were now too much like hard work, staying in one cabin and having a bit more of the world brought to us would be ideal.

Accepting that the monster called Alzheimer's was rapidly catching up I put some thought into proceeding with our wish to see as much of the world as we could. As Dave's carer, as well as his wife, I accepted (there's that word again) that whether at home or away he would have to be toileted, showered, dressed, helped to clean his teeth and assisted at meal times. There were times at home when having completed these routine duties Dave wanted immediate distraction in the form of entertainment, either days out or visitors over for lunch. How much more relaxing would it be to be able to give all care and then sit back and have wonderful meals provided, plus cabaret and all the company we needed. During what I call our 'cruising years' we certainly didn't lack company as Dave made friends so easily and when it was reciprocated by new friends seeking out our company it certainly added to my enjoyment of holidays.

In 2004 having secured a last minute deal (I was becoming adept at comparing cruise companies' prices online and by phoning cruise companies) I took Dave on a month long cruise around the East and Western Caribbean, but first we had to fly out to Fort Lauderdale USA to pick up the ship. With an overnight stay in Miami and a full day before we boarded the ship I felt apprehensive. I think that was because we had been used to being greeted and meeting up with fellow guests soon after boarding the ship, staying in a hotel in Miami even for one night made me feel vulnerable. I found the free time in Miami worrying with busy roads to cross and choosing where to eat. Dave was actually absolutely fine and I realised it was becoming more about me and my ability to manage. Once we boarded the ship and got the dreaded lifeboat drill out of the way I was alright.

The guests on the ship were predominantly American as were our neighbours on the next table who, within a couple of nights, wanted us to move our table next to theirs and join them. Having explained the situation they became even more friendly and solicitous towards Dave and added to our enjoyment with their great sense of humour. They had their problems too as one of them was almost blind. More proof that whilst it's still possible to holiday, you just have to take your problems with you. They asked us to join them on a carnival night on the top deck where brightly coloured wish balloons were given out with luggage labels attached. Everyone had written a wish on the label and they were all be released at midnight. My wish became a prayer and I can't describe the feeling of emotion I had at the sight of all those coloured balloons floating up to the Caribbean night sky. How many people aboard were desperate to have medical issues resolved and how many, not having experienced major problems in life yet, were simply wishing for things of monetary value.

Climbing into dugout canoes to visit the San Blas Islands off the coast of Panama was an experience I wouldn't want to repeat but we did it to visit people who lived very simple lives, ,or so it seemed, but like any poor part of the world their main object seemed to be to make money from the tourists. So being the cynic I am I was not happy to see two young women in colourful traditional dress bathing a baby in a hollowed out tree trunk using a tin can to pour water over his head. I hovered around fascinated as they repeated this process for photographs (yes I was guilty of taking one too). As each new group of tourists from the ship came along, into the water the baby would go again, its skin beginning to resemble a prune. In the meantime one of their other children went around collecting the dollars. The baby was crying, the tourists were muttering when suddenly a voice shouted out, 'Put some clothes on that baby'. Yes it was Dave and somehow I think he would have voiced his displeasure even if he didn't have Alzheimer's. These were very short people in stature but I admit to feeling most uncomfortable as we were on the receiving end of some scary looks as other people from the island came to join them. I couldn't wait to get back to the ship and the fact that a child was bailing out with a tin can didn't help my nerves, but what an experience. Insurance? I would think twice.

Sailing through the Panama Canal was another of Dave's ambitions realised and after we got through we were taken back to it by coach to sit in grandstand seats and watch other ships sail through so tightly that there were various colours of paint from other ships as they had squeezed their way through. I don't know if Dave appreciated the engineering feat of this anymore, but I loved the look of fascination on his face as he leaned over the ship's rail watching us squeeze through, then later on watching other ships do the same.

Halfway through the cruise many passengers disembarked and new arrivals came aboard for the other half of the cruise so the ship was fairly quiet. We were sunbathing on Deck when we were joined by Nancy from Massachusetts who I am still in touch with by e-mail to this day. Dave struck up a conversation and when it became apparent he was struggling she was so patient with him, and by the end of the afternoon we were firm friends. She had been an occupational therapist in her working life and had an immediate rapport with Dave. Her husband John used to wander around the ship with a rucksack full of books looking for a quiet space but when he did join us he had some lovely chats with Dave. Such a gentle man with a quiet sense of humour. I really do think sometimes people are put in our path to make life easier.

When we docked in St. Lucia Dave had an angry episode wanting to know where the beach was that we had seen when sailing into port. He was hot, tired, it had taken a while to disembark and it was suddenly raining heavily. The port was crowded and busy with a market and Dave thought he would be lazing on a beach and swimming in Caribbean waters. He began to shout at me incomprehensibly throwing the rucksack into a puddle when a security guard came running over, 'Hey Man, you are on vacation, just chill', he said smiling with the whitest teeth I had ever seen and with that lovely Caribbean accent. I tried to explain that Dave wasn't well and maybe we should go back to the ship but no, Dave wanted the beach. At this point the guard called over a uniformed lady taxi driver and put us in the cab bidding us to have a nice day and told her to take us to a beach. I didn't know where we were going or what it would cost (trust in God and the cab driver), but within a few minutes the rain stopped, the sun came out and she dropped us off at the clubhouse entrance to a beautiful beach telling us she would return for us in three hours and gave me an acceptable fixed price. Heaven! The only fly in the ointment was that for some reason Dave was still angry with me so while I watched him paddle around in the water I had a long cool drink watching him from the shade of a palm tree knowing he would eventually come round. This he did when we joined Nancy and John at our usual spot on the ship's deck later that afternoon. Their calming influence on him helped me to relax.

Our last port of call was Key West, where to my amazement I was approached by a friend's daughter, Jane, who was on holiday there from her home in Michigan. We hadn't met for about 15 years and we were all so excited because we had recognised one another. Dave was more excited than anyone joining in with all the hugging, but sadly, I don't really think he knew who she was.

Having finally docked in Fort Lauderdale I regarded the cruise as yet another holiday success, though I didn't relish the thought off another free day in Miami. To my surprise we were given a guided tour of Miami, taken to a recommended place for lunch and then finally escorted to the airport. Although on the flight home there were no problems I made the decision that if we were to cruise again it would not involve a flight or even a coach to a port in England.

I was later to discover that FRED OLSEN CRUISE COMPANY was sailing regularly from Liverpool and we were to become regular clients of theirs.

In 2005 we cruised to the Canary Islands and the Norwegian Fjords and from the start we got first class treatment from an amazing crew who were mainly from the Philippines, known for their smiles and friendly nature. My request for a corner table for two was granted, and after a couple of cruises we always got the same table. Dave's food was cut up for him and only the cutlery he needed was laid out. They nicknamed him Sir David and he was greeted as such when approaching the restaurant and judging by the look on some of the passengers faces I think it was believed until they heard the banter between them. We almost always sailed on 'THE BLACK PRINCE', a small ship which was less complicated. Dave would attempt deck games with the help of a very patient activity crew who in turn explained the situation to other passengers. Consequently Dave got to know many people and would warmly greet them as we walked around the deck. Sometimes I would be sitting reading my book and somebody would come and tell me where he was but I always knew he was safe. Occasionally someone would say to me, 'Aren't you afraid of him going overboard?' and I would assure them that was the last of my fears as he had absolutely no suicidal tendencies and was enjoying his holiday far too much. Of course these holidays weren't without incidents, mainly funny ones in retrospect until the last cruise of course when things weren't quite so funny anymore but there were good times ahead before that final cruise.

In 2006 we did a two week sail around Spanish ports, but I know that family and friends must have been concerned when in 2008 I booked a five week cruise to sail up the Orinoco Delta and around the Caribbean. It was a really unbelievable deal and I knew there were airports for flights home if it became a problem so decided to go ahead.

Then my lovely sister June developed cancer again. Dave and I were spending Christmas with our daughter Jane and family when we received the phone call to say June had been re-admitted to hospital on Christmas day and the family had been told she was terminally ill. Hiding my grief from Dave was hard as I knew he would be devastated. He had known her since she was only fourteen and she regarded him like a big brother.

This is another problem in being a carer; not only had I lost the emotional support and comfort from a loving caring partner but I felt I had to comfort and support him in his grief. Once again I had to be the strong one. Dave could only feel his own grief and I missed the old

Dave, the reassuring one, who would comfort and support me. I always had his love but I felt he was the one who had to be reassured, saying all the things to him that others were saying to me regarding June being free from pain.

My first instinct of course was to cancel the cruise after the Christmas holiday but when I got back from Hampshire and went to visit, although she was awake, I could see how bad things were. When Norman and their children Janet and Ian were asked to go and speak to the Consultant she held my hand and looked at me saying, 'We knew didn't we? Before I had chance to answer her family were back putting on a brave face. When leaving the hospital they fell apart as they had been told it would be weeks rather than months. We comforted one another before collecting Dave from the day room where a nurse had been chatting with him. As we were leaving she said to Dave, 'Have you lost one of your shoes?' I had taken him to the hospital with one shoe and one slipper on. That night Norman rang to say she was on oxygen and in a critical condition, so leaving Dave in the care of friends, I returned to the hospital. June died in the early hours of the following morning, 29th December, with Norman, my brother Michael and I by her bedside. I couldn't believe I had lost my little sister because that's what she would always be to me. I drove home alone at 4am in the morning with a feeling of desolation and when I climbed into bed alongside Dave he stirred and simply said, 'Has she gone?' When I replied that she had, he cried. I hadn't been sure of how much he had taken in, but now I knew.

The days that followed were difficult. The last thing I wanted to think about was the cruise but, as Norman said, what was the point of cancelling when there was nothing we could do anymore. I had Dave to think of and being in the sun for a few weeks in January would do us both good but we hadn't realised that funeral arrangements could be so delayed between Christmas and New Year. This meant the strain of waiting until the Festive season was over before knowing when the funeral would be. 'You will still be able to go', said Norman but little did we know it would be on the same day. The funeral was at 11am and the ship was to sail at 5pm with passenger boarding time at 3pm. Our friend Tom came to our aid by collecting our luggage from our home the previous evening and then picking us up from the post funeral lunch at three thirty. The embarkation staff had been told of the circumstances and allowed for a late boarding. It felt surreal arriving to board the ship with both of us smartly attired in dark clothing. Within minutes it was time for the dreaded lifeboat drill and all the confusion that entailed so after an early dinner Dave was ready for bed and soon asleep .I was left with my feelings of grief and uncertainty as to whether I had done the right thing and cried myself to sleep.

Within a couple of days I knew we had made the right decision as Dave quickly began to enjoy the sunshine we were sailing into. He also got straight into the deck games and the couple we made friends with throughout that cruise were Robert and Kathy. I had vowed I wouldn't tell anyone of June's death as I didn't want to spoil anyone's holiday but found Kathy so easy to speak to that I confided in her that we had sailed on the day of her funeral. It was like releasing a pressure valve yet we never dwelt on it again. She was so empathetic that I felt safe knowing someone else knew what I was going through. We spent so much time having a real good laugh, sharing the same sense of humour particularly at some of the incidents involving Dave. One of which was being invited to the Captain's table for dinner.

We returned to our cabin one day to find this rather ornate invitation pinned to our door and when Dave realised what it was he was delighted with this much sought after invitation. I had to burst his bubble by explaining how difficult it would be sitting with a large party of strangers making conversation. To be honest I was more concerned about my own stress levels and, although disappointed, he agreed, so I let them know at reception that we couldn't accept. At dinner that night Dave wanted to explain to the Captain personally as the Captains table was just a few feet from ours, but I dissuaded him saying that we might bump into him sometime later as he walked around the ship.

As it was a long cruise we had watched the formalities taking place as a formal photograph of Captain, officers and passengers was taken each week. Little did I know the Captain would be on top deck the following morning bird watching alongside several passengers. We were on the Orinoco River where there are some rare birds to spot. There was no stopping Dave as he approached the Captain ready to apologise for missing dinner but as it was very early in the morning Dave was struggling with his words. The Captain who was Norwegian, looked puzzled, and so I explained about Alzheimer's and he immediately said, 'I know this illness', and began to engage in conversation with Dave who told him he wanted a photo. The captain asked for someone to come and take our photo and from then on, when doing his tour of the ship, the Captain saluted Dave who of course saluted him back saying, 'Aye Aye Cap'n', and they would have a little chat. I'm sure people didn't realise how little things like that made such a difference to Dave's enjoyment.

Sunbathing on a beautiful beach a few days later the cabaret singer from the ship arrived and settled down for some rest and relaxation. She had already waved and said hello having recognised us from the ship (Dave was hard to ignore). He wanted her to have his sunbed as she was only lying on a towel, but she explained that she only had an hour and that's why she hadn't hired one. Dave was determined to engage her in conversation so I explained the situation, suggesting she may like to move somewhere quieter but in fact she moved nearer and seemed happy to enjoy Dave's company. She'd had some experience in her family with dementia so as a result of our chance meeting on the beach she became another one of Dave's cruising buddies. Every show she did, as she took a bow, she would come over to where we were sitting and plant a kiss on Dave's cheek to his delight. Someone asked me if she was she a relative and I had to say that she wasn't, but just one of my husband's many girlfriends and such a glamorous one at that.

The holiday was a great success and so we continued cruising for another four years from Liverpool .We did a Baltic cruise, which involved visiting St Petersburg and going to a Russian Ballet Company to see a performance of Giselle. On entering the theatre all the programme sellers were in the most beautiful coloured crinoline gowns so Dave was enthralled before the ballet even started. The Black Prince also took us to Croatia and Venice where we had another evening of culture sailing up to the most beautiful theatre for a musical evening. None of these cruises were without incidents and every time I came home I would say, 'I don't think I can do this anymore', but I don't regret one of them.

On one of the Black Prince Cruises around ports of Spain I felt comfortable about Dave wandering around such a small ship as he usually stayed within my view. It could be a bit embarrassing when he went on to the upper sun deck, leaned on the rail and hollered, 'Joan', at the top of his voice, but people soon got to know him. One afternoon he asked if he could go to the indoor pool on his own. It was pretty straightforward, on the same deck we were on, so I walked him there and having already got his swim shorts on left his towel, T shirt and shorts over a rail near the men's changing room (he was still able to dress at this point) when it was just shorts at this point. I went back to reading my book, but after a few minutes I couldn't settle so went to watch him swim. His wet swim shorts were hanging over the rail, his towel was gone but his clothes were still near the changing room. 'Are you looking for Dave?' called the only man swimming in the pool.

When I replied that I was he said, 'He's only just got out but I think he's gone over to the Sauna'.

I collected his clothes and as I entered the changing room area I heard a lady's querulous voice shouting, 'Has he gone, has he gone?' Opening the door to a cubicle I found Dave cowering with his towel around him looking really worried.

'You've not got your clothes Dave', I said when, from a partition behind him, appeared a little white haired elderly lady with a green face mask on, her eyes staring out of her little green face. I apologised and tried to explain Dave's confusion but all she could say was,

'Take him away, take him away', he shouldn't be allowed'. Taking him in to the nearest ladies' toilet I got him dressed realising that he was as scared as she was. 'Her face was green', he kept saying. Walking him back to the cabin I reassured him and we both saw the funny side of it when I explained it was a face mask. At dinner that night I couldn't help teasing him a little as every white haired lady walked in I asked, 'Do you think it was her Dave?' As long as she didn't recognise him he saw the funny side but that was the last time he went anywhere alone on the ship.

I always waited until the ship was almost empty before going ashore unless we had an organised trip. By doing this there were less crowds and Dave would know we were just going to get on the shuttle bus when most of the other passengers were gone. We were sitting waiting one day when Dave started a conversation with a lady called Ida who had an immediate rapport with him. She was someone else with experience caring for people with dementia so it was relaxing to sit quietly while waiting to go ashore. When her husband Bobby joined us I asked if we were keeping them back, but they explained they had been to this particular port many times as he worked on the ship. Dave asked what he did and when told he was Bobby Kaye the ship's comedian Dave said, 'You can't be him. He's got red hair. I remember you'. There was a series of television programme in the sixties called THE COMEDIANS and Bobby made many appearances on it and is still well known and loved on the club circuit. Because it was so long since we'd seen him I hadn't recognised him either but, here was Dave disputing it. Dave went to look at the photo advertising his show and came back saying, 'You've got red hair on that photo'.

'It's an old photo', said Bobby laughing. I think Bobby liked that publicity photo because he had hair then but he is now what you would call follicly challenged. As a result of our conversation that morning we spent many times having a real good laugh when he wasn't on stage. He introduced us to another couple they had made friends when their father was with them and who also had dementia. We had some confusing conversations at times but really enjoyed each other's company and when Bobby was on stage we had to have front row seats, although I was always a bit wary of Dave joining in his act.

Most cruises on the Black Prince had a similar itinerary but that didn't matter to us as we were on it for the convenience of sailing from Liverpool. Each cruise told a story of one of Dave's mishaps. We once met a Scottish couple from Jerusalem and again we struck up a friendship. Edwin couldn't hide his admiration for the way Dave was carrying on trying to live and enjoy as normal a life as possible. He also got quite emotional to the point of tears when Dave and I stumbled around the dance floor for a waltz or a jive.

We docked in Malta one day and Edwin and Doreen took us to meet an old friend from Dental College who owned a couple of shops on the main street. They hadn't seen one another for about fifty years but on introduction Dave chatted to this old friend of theirs as though he knew him well and had only seen him last week.

Whist in Malta we had the usual minor dispute regarding the buying of souvenirs and, of course, Dave couldn't understand that to keep having holidays meant watching what we spent but he never wanted anything cheap, other than another of one of his beloved baseball hats. This time it was an icon of the Holy Family, because of his strong faith in God, which never wavered even when things got really tough. So there we were looking in a jeweller's window with Edwin saying, 'Joan, he's got to have that'. Although belonging to the Jewish Faith he could see how much this meant to Dave. So, like the expensive crystal emu from New Zealand which he created such a fuss about until I bought it, I had to give in and buy it. The Plaque of the Holy family is now one of my treasures standing at the side of my bed with a holiday photo of Dave, with a huge smile on his face.

The main memory of that particular cruise was Dave falling into the swimming pool with all his clothes on. We had been walking around the ship with Edwin and Doreen, and as it was late afternoon, the sun was going down at the back of the ship so we decided to sit and watch. To get there meant negotiating some steps but Dave was refusing to hold my hand and was making his own way but getting nearer to the pool. I skirted around it with all three of us warning, 'Dave, you are going to fall in', or words to that effect when suddenly there was a huge splash as in he went. I ran around to the pool steps but when he surfaced I don't know whether it was embarrassment or sheer stubbornness on his part but he behaved as though, this was no accident; this is what he meant to do he said. He came up for air, baseball hat at a jaunty angle and his puffa jacket looking a lot more puffed up than when he went in; he looked just like the Michelin man in the adverts. I was calling for him to swim to the steps as he just floated on his back smiling and saying how lovely it was. We were on the way home and it wasn't lovely, it was cold but even when a passenger dived in to help he refused to be helped saying, 'You're alright mate, I'm fine'. When we finally got him to come out he was one dripping soggy mess and as there was a ladies changing room nearby I had to strip him off, wrap him in towels and leave him with Edwin and Doreen while I dashed back to the cabin for a set of clothes. The alternative would have been to march him through the ship's lounge during afternoon tea wrapped in towels; now wouldn't that have caused a stir! When I finally got him dressed and back in the cabin he immediately fell asleep so I took the opportunity to go to the lounge for a coffee. While I was sitting there a man turned and said to me, 'Did you know a man with Alzheimer's fell in the pool just before. I wonder why no one was watching him'. I explained that he was being watched but it still happened. Then I just relaxed with my coffee. Sometimes it's just too tiring to explain. Dave was no worse for wear and thought it funny when we talked about it the next day. In fact I think he was quite proud of being the man who fell in to the pool.

On that cruise we also met Betty from Yorkshire who we had met on a previous cruise. She was a real character and as Dave approached her with open arms I wasn't sure if he recognised her or not (he was still great at bluffing). Having lunch with her one day she could see he was struggling and embarrassed about food spillage. Diving into her handbag she said, 'Now I know how I can help you here Dave because being a lady with an ample bosom, I often make a bit of a mess', and with that she produced a beaded chain with clips on either end which she attached to her linen napkin. 'There' she said, 'that's much better'. It saves the napkin sliding down my front'. Quite casually she produced another one saying, 'Here Dave let me put this on you', and he willingly accepted her help. I thought I had seen most aids and told her I sometimes put a tea towel around his neck but found them too bulky.

'Well' she said, 'I was in the dentist's one day and he put this contraption around my neck and I though that's just the job, so I told him I was going on a cruise and he let me have a couple'. Good old Betty from Yorkshire and thank you Andrew the dentist.

Farewell to the Black Prince 2009

All good things must come to an end so it was with sadness I heard that the Black prince was to sail on her final voyage and how ironic to realise towards the end of that cruise it would also be our final voyage. She had been sailing since 1966 and it was to be her final voyage in October 2009. Although Dave had worsened in many ways I still felt we could cope but would have to pay extra for a bigger cabin and bathroom with a bath so I could stand him in it, with room to shower him.

I took a chance on how he would be nearer the time and booked. Cabins would be much sought after as it was the last cruise. Most regular passengers on the ship regarded it as a family or club at sea and we witnessed many reunions of passengers from previous cruises and although problems had increased Dave fully understood and was eager to go on this cruise which was to be to Iceland and then around Great Britain.

On embarkation sure enough we recognised many faces and the reunions started before we left Liverpool.

Paying for a bigger cabin and booking early didn't solve our problems though, as although we had a bigger bathroom using the toilet meant opening the door inwards and standing to the side of the sink before closing it revealing the toilet behind the door. It was a real struggle, if I went in first I couldn't manoeuvre Dave in behind me and, if I got him in first he would stand to the side of the sink looking puzzled. So it was either use the disabled toilet on deck, or during the night or early morning, allow him to use the bath and then clean up afterwards. Bathing or showering wasn't much better as there wasn't enough room for me to get him out and dry; consequently by the time I got him to his bed where his clothes were laid out he wasn't in a very good humour. By the time we got to breakfast though the crew could always change his mood, saying, 'Good morning Sir David', and escorting him to our table. Although breakfast was self-service the help they gave me was amazing, Knowing Dave would follow me if I left the table they bought our juice and cereal to us and then hovered around Dave while I went to the grill. Without Fred Olsen's crew on various ships we would never have been able to continue having holidays, meeting all those wonderful people and keeping a sense of normality in our lives. I say 'we' because without doubt the effect on both of us as the illness progressed was devastating at times.

It seemed to take longer to settle on this cruise and I admit to feeling concerned and a little stressed at times, wondering about what I'd done. Had I pushed things too far and made a huge mistake? But we just took it one day at a time and when we saw the wild scenery and amazing geezers in Iceland, shooting up hot steaming water, to see Dave's excitement at this sight made it so worthwhile.

That cruise was so different as we saw parts of the U.K. that were wild and beautiful, such as the Hebrides and the Shetland Isles where we took a local bus to Scalloway, which was freezing, and visited the museum learning about the heroic deeds concerning 'The Shetland Bus', which returned refugees from German occupied Norway to the Shetlands. Listening to the curator I thought most of this information would go over Dave's head but he was really interested, particularly when we heard that one of the heroes was an old boy of our grandson Matthew's school. So of course Dave insisted we buy the book about his heroism.

Another wild and wonderful place that I had always wanted to see was The Giants Causeway in Northern Ireland and it was (to use my grandchildren's expression) awesome. Dave's coordination wasn't very good when trying to negotiate slippery rocks but it was so worth it. A sunny day but with gusts of wind that nearly blew us off our feet; this cruise was not for wimps.

Our Final Cruise on the Boudica 2009 :

The last formal evening two nights before we disembarked from the 2010 Western Mediterranean made me realise our cruising days were over.

Although personal care was not easy Dave loved the formality of dressing for dinner and as time went on I made adjustments e.g. black trousers with elasticated waist to go with his dinner jacket, and bow tie with elastic so it could be slipped over his head. He would stand and admire the finished result in the mirror often saying, 'I do look so posh don't I?' On any given evening Dave liked to make an entrance and then wander around speaking to people and as the guests around us on that cruise were particularly friendly I would sit down until he was ready to join me. There was a table to the right of our corner table with a party of eight ladies and another party of four immediately behind Dave, where a mother and three daughters, were celebrating the mum's birthday. He would ask them if everything was alright and how was everybody behaving, like a self-appointed maître'd. That last evening was like any other except that he was a little slower at coming back to our table and when he did I knew by the expression on his face that things weren't right as he was giving me the most surly looks. Sure enough when his first course came he started to pick up pieces of smoked salmon, looking at it with disgust and then throwing it towards me saying, 'What's this supposed to be?' I sent the first course back hoping we would be better with the main meal but he got up and started going walkabout speaking to people further away and shouting at me when I tried to get him to come back. The only thing to do was to leave the restaurant and persuade him to come with me, but things became physical when he began to twist my arm. Security were called and even though they handled things in a sensitive manner I could feel his mood worsening. Then along came Tony from Yorkshire (Yorkshire to the rescue again) who very casually tried to intervene. Dave seemed bewildered but smiled at Tony as he and the security man escorted us back to the cabin, but I was public enemy number one and catching sight of me seemed to flare him up again. I felt absolutely sick as I opened the cabin door and let Tony bring him in. I had never envisaged anything as sudden as this, and even though it had happened at home it had never happened so badly and in such a public place, and to be at sea was terrifying. I got some nightwear out and managed to persuade Dave to take a Diazepam, the only time I had needed to do this so far on the cruise. Tony was amazing with him; one minute they were having a sing-along and the next Dave was swearing and shouting at him, but if I appeared he went berserk. So I stayed outside the cabin and was joined by the ship's doctor, nurse and security man who were all concerned for my safety. I assured the doctor that I had all the prescribed medication Dave needed and that he would settle down eventually. I wish I had felt as confident inside but I was scared stiff. Eventually Tony came out saying Dave appeared to have drifted off but to send someone for him if I needed help. The fact was that I had never even met Tony until that night. I had seen him and his wife around the ship but never spoken to him yet that night he really was my saviour; another person I will never forget. The nurse said that after discussion with the doctor they would feel happier if I would sit outside the cabin door for a couple of hours until he really settled, and somebody from security would walk passed every 20 minutes or so. I also promised I would ring the emergency number during the night if necessary. I managed to sneak in and get a chair and my book and, as they were aware I had missed dinner, they arranged for a tray to be sent from the galley even though food was the last thing on my mind. So there I was on our last formal evening sitting outside my Cabin in my gorgeous, sparkly, formal evening gown reading my book and eating sandwiches and chips. As people passed by returning to their cabins I simply glanced up and gave them a smiling goodnight as though all was well with the world but I can't explain the feeling of doom I felt inside. It wasn't just about the last cruise or holiday it was about the final stage of Alzheimer's Disease rapidly approaching. The following morning I was awake before Dave and watched for his facial expression to see if, as often happened, he would remember and be upset, but I could see he was still angry looking. So, deciding to forego the shower routine, I used wet wipes and got him dressed as quickly as I could, all the time assuring him that everything was going to be alright and how glad I was he was feeling better and that he was doing so well. I was just rambling really and wasn't sure how the day would pan out. Taking him to the snack café I got toast for us both rather than risk the restaurant. We spent the morning strolling around the ship keeping away from people as I felt the less stimulus the better.

There was a piano recital of light classical music in the afternoon which he always enjoyed so as the day went on he relaxed, but didn't mention events of the night before. Yet in the evening we went to the show and he spotted Tony in the audience saying, 'There's that man who helped us last night, can we buy him a drink?' I asked the waiter to get a drink for him and his wife on my ship's card and Dave waved to him vigorously shouting his thanks. At the end of the evening everyone joined hands for Auld Lang Syne and many tears were shed as emotional farewells were made on this final cruise but I had to keep my emotions in check for a very different reason.

When we began to disembark the following morning I was a little concerned as Dave seemed subdued and nervous not letting go of my hand so I left the luggage in the customs shed and went out to find brother in law Paul who was coming to take us home. After collecting our luggage Paul realised that Dave didn't recognise him at all so I sat in the back of the car with Dave. The journey home only took half an hour and Paul said that when he got home to Barbara, Dave's sister, he was disturbed about it and told her that Dave wasn't himself and hadn't recognised him.

A few days at home and things settled down but without being able to explain how, things were now different. This cruel disease is insidious, it takes away the person little by little and sort of creeps up on you giving you a jolt now and then just in case you think you are getting away with it and daring to behave like other people do.

We still kept up with our support group meetings but he was becoming a little less extrovert. At some of the meetings he had danced, shaking maracas with Julian (who has also since died, sadly) or with the Morris dancers one of whom, was Jeanette, his nurse. He was famous for announcing himself, 'It is I', and our grandchildren loved his random sayings like, 'Rhubarb and 'roll over'. He still tried so hard but conversation, which had always been difficult, was becoming one sided with Dave offering only the odd sentence. 'Is there anyone in this house?' was a favourite, even when I was in the same room. As was, 'JOAN!' at the top of his voice when I was right there. The neighbours heard that one regularly as well as, 'Why do you do this?' or 'Has something happened?' when he was anxious. Of course there was always the, 'Why am I posh?' when we were going out anywhere, and I learnt to judge whether he was anxious or happy about going out by the tone in which he said this.

I knew holidays, as we had known them, were over and accepted this as we had been flying by the seat of our pants for quite some time. I have absolutely no regrets about all the travelling we did, meeting people from all over the world who are still in touch with us. I know from what they tell me that he left a massive impression on them. Now socialising, which had been respite for me, was not as pleasurable for either of us. I couldn't relax and felt I was on guard duty watching for any problems that might arise.

Some things he did really made us chuckle, but not in front of him. There was the time when we were visiting Jane, Paul and the children and after watching Jane grooming the dog Pippin as he played with his sheepskin blanket, Dave asked if he could do it. Thinking it would be relaxing and quite therapeutic Jane gave him the grooming comb only to come back and find the dog had gone and Dave was combing the rug.

So 2010 and 2011 were quite different. We still went to the safari park but he wasn't focussing and we could have been driving along on a normal road; he wasn't enjoying himself as much. We went to the cinema less. He couldn't cope with busy places. Our friends and family were just as supportive, inviting us for meals etc but, particularly when we were alone, there was very little to say. Meaningful conversations had become a thing of the past. He always perked up when the family came home though; Sophie with her boisterous teasing which always made him laugh and as for the younger girls Millie, Annie and Jess, well he would have been content to sit on the couch all day and accept their cuddles. He was in awe of how tall Matthew had become and constantly said to me and anyone who cared to listen, 'He's such a lovely boy, you know', and he still liked to do short walks around the block with all of them. Also his Brother Derek and Sister Barbara were still very much involved and I knew if it was a tough day they would be there at the drop of a hat on top of their regular visits.

Chapter 23

DAVE'S 70th BIRTHDAY

August 8th 2011 was an important time as it was Dave's 70th birthday and we were all hoping he would be well enough to celebrate it with a big party for family and friends at our local club St Mary's Birchley. The club where he had helped to run a youth disco, played Santa at the pensioner's party, worked the entertainment lights for Saturday night dances and where we held our Ruby wedding party the year after he was diagnosed. As the time approached I was aware of changes almost every day but when all the family arrived at the weekend he was so excited and I really do think he knew it was a big occasion.

The family went on ahead to decorate the club lounge and when I got him there, 'all posh' as he said, he was well aware that it was all about him when he saw all the balloons, banners and display of photo's from yesteryear. As people began to arrive he became more and more excited and I did worry there might be too much stimulus but he seemed to take it all in his stride. That was until 'ELVIS' arrived. Yes, we had booked a tribute act. This Elvis had appeared at a MIND party the year before and Dave had absolutely loved him, so I had managed to track him down.

Apart from family and friends his guests included friends with Alzheimer's and their carers, Dave's past and present carers, Jeanette his nurse, people from

MIND and Joan, Carol and Jane from 'Making Sense'; all there to help him celebrate his big day. He loved all the attention and I was aware that at times he was becoming a bit over excited but when Elvis came on in his white spangled suit singing 'Love Me Tender' Dave was completely enraptured. We both had seats immediately in front of this wonderful entertainer who knew the situation and involved Dave and I from the word go. If it was a slow song he got us up to waltz and anything faster Dave needed no encouragement to do a bit of moving and shaking sometimes preparing to launch himself at Elvis.

One of the guests said her funniest memory was of Dave eagerly shuffling his seat forward in his excitement and me, desperately holding on to his belt trying to keep him sitting down for at least some of the act. Turning Dave's collar up Elvis style the Entertainer placed an Elvis style emerald green scarf around his neck and Dave thought he was the bees knees. There was great hilarity when Elvis got our daughter Jane, her friend Leslie and our friends Howard and Peter up to take part in a hip swivelling competition to 'Rock-a-Hula Baby'.

When the buffet was served I got us a table and instead of going back into the lounge with everyone else stayed with close family encouraging him to eat and have a cold drink. He needed to chill out for a while before becoming a party animal again. What a surprise when we did enter the lounge as our granddaughters, Millie and Jessica, had brought their violins and Annie, who didn't play, had brought the bongo drums to keep time.

They had been rehearsing 'Happy Birthday', and were all set up in the corner of the lounge with their music stands. Quiet was called for as they played for their lovely granddad. You could have heard a pin drop as they played, with Dave sat immediately in front of them. So many guests said later they felt so emotional with tears in their eyes.

The day ended with copies of the song 'Always look On the Bright side of Life' being passed around and everyone joined in whole heartedly. I've never seen so many smiling faces. Dave was able to say his goodbyes and thank everyone for coming, this time knowing it really had been all about him. This had been the only birthday in years he hadn't celebrated with our friend Arthur but, as it was Arthur's 70th too, Pat had surprised him with the birthday gift of a cruise around the Hebrides. Ironically Dave hadn't remembered that they had always shared birthdays or noticed that they weren't there even though we regularly looked at photographs of past birthday parties and holidays. This made me realise that living life one day at a time was becoming increasingly important for Dave. Yesterday is past and tomorrow may never come so all we have is today, the present, and a present is a gift to be enjoyed a day at a time .

Chapter 24

AUGUST TO CHRISTMAS 2011

As time went on there were changes almost on a daily basis and it wasn't as easy to distract or keep him occupied. It was the aggression I feared most so I learned to listen to his tone of voice and watch his facial expression to judge the mood he was in, but I wasn't always able to do much about it. That insight into his own illness never left him and the part I found most heart-breaking was when I walked into the room and, without making a sound he would be sitting there quietly with tears rolling down his cheeks.

'What's the matter Dave?' I would say as sympathetically as I could (what a stupid question).

He would just shake his head in despair. Or sometimes he would get up and walk to the window, look out of it and say, 'I want to go Joan', and I knew exactly what he meant. I had exhausted all distraction techniques and looking back I think depression may have been setting in. I felt an overwhelming sense of sadness at what seemed to be the futility of it all but instead of trying to cheer him up it was enough to sit holding hands and just say, 'It's not bloody fair'. Being the amazingly brave person he was he would see what it was doing to me and pull himself together saying, 'Onward and upward'.

I never envisaged him going into residential care. I had always planned he would stay home with me until the end. Friends were beginning to comment that I was looking tired and I admit to wondering occasionally how long I could do this, mainly if we had an aggressive episode. Whatever happened Sue and Jane had told me they were right behind me in whatever decision was made. What I did do was arrange for another night of respite care at Kavanagh Place knowing he would be in good hands with carers who loved him.

I would like to say that he always went there willingly but sadly that wasn't always so and that's when the bogey man of guilt came to haunt me again. I would tell him where we were going, he would appear to understand and then when we reached a particular part of the East Lancashire Road he knew what was happening and his breathing would become irregular and he would become tearful. I would talk him around telling him that I was tired and this was a way of keeping him at home for the rest of the week.

'I know, I know, ok', he would say, and make an effort to relax and sing to the sixties cd we had on. He was wonderful the way he tried so hard to convince me he was alright and I absolutely hated having to do this but I so needed the respite.

Once we got there and he settled it was fine and I could drive home for a relaxing weekend. Once, Karen one of the nurses rang me saying, 'Joan, I know this sounds strange but Dave has got it into his head that you are dead and I think the only way to reassure him is to speak to him'.

He came on to the phone and I assured him I was alive and well and would be coming for him the following day.

'Oh Thank God for that', was the response. 'Are you sure you are ok?' Once he knew all was well he was fine. He had probably dozed off and had a bad dream. I could hear the relief in his voice and thank goodness Karen had rung and let me speak to him rather than try to placate him. What kind of confusing thoughts must have been running around that tired brain of his. If life is hard being a carer imagine how much harder it must be living in all that confusion. Not every person suffering dementia is sitting in a pleasantly confused state, some like Dave are tormented, but thank God that was only towards the end.

One of the gifts he had received for his birthday from Jane, Paul and the girls was to spend a weekend in the Trough of Bowland in Lancashire. It was an area we knew well and when Sue and Jane were children we often took a trip there for the day and enjoyed picnics and walks. They had booked a National Trust cottage and although the weather wasn't great when we got there we enjoyed a lovely meal together in the farmhouse style kitchen. The following day we did a short walk on a good footpath that actually passed the front door. Jane and Paul were able to do a much longer walk with the dog, Pippin, while we enjoyed some quality time with the girls. Just chilling out as they would say. In the afternoon we revisited Dunsop Bridge, a particular favourite spot where we had been many times with Dave's mum. I wondered if being there would evoke any memories for Dave but as usual if I said, 'Do you remember?'……. He just agreed. Visiting Chipping nearby, famous for its ice cream, also took us down memory lane but I couldn't tell if Dave remembered or not. It certainly was a great day out though, rain or no rain.

As thoughts of Christmas began I knew it would be more difficult that year even though transport wasn't a problem, as instead of the train journey (which I knew was now out of the question) we had a lift with Jane's mother and father in-law. Sue, Wayne and family were back from Singapore and living in Guilford, which was a forty minute drive from Jane and Paul's in Hampshire. The plan was to travel to Jane's where we would be collected by Sue a couple of hours later, spend Christmas Eve and Day with Sue and family and then all go back to Jane, Paul and Co for a Boxing Day buffet and have all the family together. Although I had explained all the plans to Dave he became confused. It was all too much but the journey down was fine; we stopped at the services and he laughed and joked with John. He was always alright with Hilda as she was one of his ladies he had a special soft spot for. When we arrived he was happy to see everyone and played with Annie, Millie and the dog, Pippin.

When Sue arrived with Jessica he was even more pleased to see all his girls together, so I began to relax and think it would all work out well.

After saying goodbye to everyone we set off for Guilford just as it was beginning to go dark. There were soon signs of agitation as Dave repeatedly asked where we were going. He was sitting in the back of the car with Jessica and she constantly tried to reassure him that he was going to have a lovely Christmas, but as we drove through the centre of Guilford his agitation became worse. Fortunately our destination was just outside the city. As we drove up the drive there was a note of panic in Dave's voice as he said, 'What is this place, where are we?'.

We had only been to the house once before since they came back from Singapore, so between the newness of it all and his recent deterioration I began to get a feeling of foreboding. However, as soon as Dave was greeted by Sue's husband Wayne, and Matthew and Sophie, he seemed to get on a more level footing and we all had a wonderful Christmas Eve dinner, but I felt an early night would be helpful.

The following morning, as Christmas Day dawned, he looked a little bewildered as we could hear Jess going down to open her presents with Matthew and Sophie soon following . We joined the rest of the family and Dave really did appear to get into the spirit of Christmas but then problems arose after breakfast as he kept squeezing my hand and asking, 'Where are we?' and, 'When are we going?' Sue kept reassuring me that everything was alright but I could sense Dave was going to go out of control and admit I was afraid that we would spoil Christmas for everyone. Taking him into another room I explained again where we were and that it was Christmas so we didn't want to spoil it for the grandchildren, how hard Sue was working to give us a nice time etc and managed to persuade him to take a Diazepam. I really think he thought we had brought him to another care home as it was such a big house and one he wasn't familiar with. He had said once or twice recently, 'I'm going to have to go away Joan. This is all too much'. His insight into his own illness never left him. Looking out of the window I pointed out Sue and Wayne's cars on the drive, and the other houses belonging to their neighbours and gradually as the Diazepam took effect, we sat quietly on the couch and he became reassured and more relaxed. I appealed to him to try extra hard for the children's sake and bless him he kept nodding saying, 'I will Joan, I will'.

So we had a lovely Christmas dinner after all and later in the afternoon went for a short walk with Sophie, which I felt helped him get his bearings a little more. As evening approached I sensed him becoming unsettled again, so knowing how tired he must be, I suggested he go to bed, which he readily agreed to, but only if I went too. I went up and stayed with him until he drifted off, but as I tried to leave he woke and asked me to stay, so I settled myself on a chair with my book. Sue kept coming up to see if we were ok and suggesting I go down for a while but I was fine. Christmas day had turned out to be lovely after all. I had felt so nervous about how Dave was going to be that morning so an early night was no problem. Anything positive was a bonus those days.

The following afternoon and overnight was to be spent at Jane and Pauls, where we would have all the family together so, after a lazy morning, we set off for their house. Dave seemed less confused as he chatted to the grandchildren. Arriving there of course meant an increase in the number of people but he chatted with everyone and played with the dog and, of course, he had his lovely daughters together whom he adored. He was pleased to see Hilda and john, but immediately associated them with going home and so began to ask again when we were going. I explained that Jane had prepared a Boxing Day party for us all before we left (I would tackle bedtime later).

I felt quite calm and confident at first and as we moved in to the conservatory he sat by Hilda for a while chatting but, as I put some food on his plate the look he gave was unmistakeable and directed at me. I could see his mood beginning to change but this time instead of appearing agitated and nervous he began to look angry. He suddenly jumped up shouting, 'I'm off!' just as he would at home when he had a need to get out quickly. The difference was that Jane's house was off the beaten track a couple of miles from a decent footpath or road and with no street lighting he would have fallen into a ditch or walked into the path of any oncoming car. I immediately followed him to the door followed by Sue and Jane, and as I tried to stop him opening the door he became more angry, twisting my fingers.

Sue tried to persuade him to wait and let her get her boots on so she could go out with him, but then he made for the stairs and the front bedroom where he proceeded to look for an escape route via the bedroom window or even the wardrobe at one point. The girls have certainly never heard such colourful language from their father before and, as most of it seemed to be directed at me, they asked if I would go out of the room and let them handle things.

I stood outside heartbroken as I heard them pleading , cajoling ,trying anything to calm him down. I stood outside, Diazepam at the ready and as things seemed to escalate I went in to try and persuade him to take his medication, all to no avail. He had launched Jane at the window and twisted her arm and was now battling with Sue to get at the window again. At one point Sue suggested they said the 'Our father', something he did at home when he felt a rage coming on, but this time he wasn't for praying.

He did eventually take the tablet but continued to rage. We were all exhausted and there was no sign of it abating. At one point I stood in the doorway watching Sue struggle as Dave cried bitterly. 'Do you think it's time to call for professional help?' I asked her.
'I was just thinking that mum', she said. I was loathe to do this as I knew what the implications might be .

We had already asked Wayne, Paul and John to allow us to try and manage Dave on our own, as the more people who became involved the more violent he might become. We were at the other end of the country so we would have had to call the emergency services, which would probably have involved the police who, through no fault of their own, would not have known how to handle Dave other than by restraining him and the result would have been Dave being sectioned under the Mental Health Act. My worst nightmare!

He was so hot and suddenly his knees began to buckle through sheer exhaustion. We were all exhausted as he lay there crying but fighting to get up now and then, as though sleep meant giving in. We persuaded him to let us help him off with his sweater so that he could have a rest with his t shirt and pants on but didn't have to go to sleep. Of course he did eventually drop off and slept through the night through sheer exhaustion. So that was the end of our Boxing Day party after all those preparations. Sue and her family went home soon after and I think we all knew that Christmas would never be the same again as far as their dad and granddad was concerned. The strange part about Dave's behaviour, as I lay in bed reflecting on the events of the day, was that, at one point he ran from upstairs to downstairs and back in an extremely agitated state, ignoring the adults and the grandchildren, yet pausing to pat Pippin the dog saying, 'Hia mate'.

The following morning it was apparent that he knew the night before had been traumatic, and as Jane helped him to eat his Weetabix, with each spoonful he took he kept saying, 'I'm so sorry love'.

'You have nothing to be sorry for dad', she said

On our journey home the following day although traffic was slow moving there were no long hold ups, thank goodness, as it was a long drive for John and the motorway was always a nightmare the day after Boxing Day. I had never had a problem with the toilets on motorway services before but this time the disabled toilet was inside the ladies or gents and, as there was a queue at the ladies I had to take Dave into the gent's disabled toilet, by which time it was too late as he couldn't hold on any longer. I had to tie his big jacket around his waist to get him to the car. I felt life shift a little more as I realised that from now on I would have to take a spare set of clothes whenever we went anywhere. The one thing that it took me almost to the end to accept was that he was becoming incontinent. Although I was toileting him every two hours at home I was always looking for a reason as to why if he had an accident, usually blaming myself for not getting him there in time.

So that was Christmas 2011 done and dusted and leaving me quite low as I tried to come to terms with this horrendous disease as it progressed. 'OK, Mr Alzheimer's,' I thought, 'You're winning; you're wearing me down and taking him from me.' Then during that week he settled down, listening to his music and watching Les Miserables. New Year was coming and so were the children and grandchildren. Jane, Paul and the girls arrived first on New Year's E,ve with the dog of course. Sue, Wayne and co would come on New Year's Day after spending the Eve with Wayne's parents and the rest of his family. We had always spent New Year's Eve with all of our friends at Marj and Jim's. It used to be fancy dress and some of the outfits were unbelievable, and then, as we had all become a little more sedate over the years (not really) we changed it to dinner suits, glam dresses and fireworks at midnight. Even if Jane and family weren't coming I knew I couldn't risk our friend's party. After the events of Christmas I realised that crowded rooms were to be avoided as there was too much stimulus.

We had a very pleasant dinner and afterwards Dave played with the dog and cuddled the girls (or the other way round), and then at about nine thirty Dave announced he was going to bed. It was no use explaining that it was a special night. He was tired, one day had now become much the same as another to him, so we settled him down and Jane lay on the bed with him just chatting. I went up to see him later and as I walked around the bed to sit on the chair he held his hand out and with a broad smile on his face he said, 'Here she is, she's always been the girl for me'. I joked about how it took him two years to ask me out from when I first met him and he said, 'No, I always knew'.

He was in a lovely mood and an hour later he was back downstairs in his dressing gown in time for Auld Lang Syne. So there we were Dave, Jane, Paul ,Millie, Annie and myself not forgetting Pippin, making a circle and singing the New Year in.   I couldn't help that surge of hope that maybe things would settle down and we would get away with it for a little while longer. This euphoric feeling stayed with me and I felt it was the best New Year's Eve I had ever had.

The following day Sue and family arrived and once again Dave thoroughly enjoyed the company of Matt, Sophie and Jessica as he watched them interact with their cousins. He really was on good form as he relaxed with just the family.

So we were into January 2012 and on the 4th Pat and Arth had a get together and we ordered a Chinese take away. I set a place at the table for Dave and helped him with his food and, although he acknowledged everyone, they had to come to him and there was no wandering around greeting people as he had done did in the past. As soon as I saw signs of tiredness we left.

January 25th was our Alzheimer's support group's belated Christmas meal in Larkins, a very casual family run restaurant which we had frequented for years. We had a whole room to ourselves making it very homely. Dave really did enjoy that day, blowing kisses to Denise the group leader, starting sing-alongs before we had even got to the end of the meal. When it came to going home he and Harry, who also had Alzheimer's, both found it hilarious as Brenda his wife and I struggled to get them into the car.

My birthday was on the 29th of January. They had helped him make a card for me at Kavanagh Place and with some prompting he wished me Happy Birthday, and also told me he loved me and that I was beautiful. He always commented without prompting when I was dressed up for a special occasion. How many 69 year olds were constantly told they were beautiful?

Dave was on form that day and anyone would have thought he was just a larger than life character. He danced, sang at the drop of a hat and had Mark in stitches laughing. Barry wore a male (chauvinistic) apron with the female body form on the front (blow up boobs with tassels included). Dave, without any prompting repeatedly went up to Barry squeezing the boobs and making a honking sound but trying to keep a straight face. It was a great , happy day and I could feel myself being lulled into a false sense of security thinking, perhaps that this year's not going to be so bad after all; perhaps he just wasn't well at Christmas.

February 1st, we went to Marie and Joe's for lunch and he knew who they were and coped very well. We also went to Marj and Jim's a couple of weeks later for lunch and to watch a Cliff Richard DVD, where once again he was on good form singing and dancing along to Cliff. That was significant because it was the last time I was able to accept a social invitation which included both of us, as another downward spiral was about to produce a rapid decline.

Dave's mood swings became worse but what distressed me more than that was the silence as tears rolled down his cheeks on the days when there was no distracting him. Doreen from Crossroads Care continued to come but had had to ring me twice to come home before I had even driven into town . On the second occasion he had frightened her by grabbing her by the scarf around her neck and when I got home he refused to speak to either of us.We both acknowledged that he was getting worse and Jeanette, his Community Psychiatric Nurse began to notice a difference.

I still had the support of family and friends, thank God, which brought some normality into a life which was becoming more and more difficult as I was now accepting that I might have to stay in with any carers.

It was important that I maintained contact with friends old and new. I did manage a reunion lunch with some of the girls who I had worked with on the same ward for almost twenty years, and also with the girls with whom I had studied for my 'Diploma for the Care of Children with Special Needs', two years before I retired. We had a meal arranged for February 24th. I can remember feeling so relaxed as it was on a Friday night and as Dave was at Kavanagh Place there was little chance of my mobile going off. I think that night as I drove home I acknowledged for the first time the thought that I could have this freedom more often if Dave went into residential care.

The staff at Kavanagh Place often passed comment that they didn't know how I coped and I began to take notice of what they were saying. Yet between all this mayhem I still had the most loving caring man who deserved all the love and care I could give. As I often said to him, 'You would do it for me, ' and he would have done. He also still had this amazing insight into his own deteriorating condition and I just wanted to take the fear away.

Would you believe that at the beginning of March he began to ask about holidays when looking through a brochure one day and I defiantly thought, why not? We could go to Southport which is only a half hour drive away. There had been a new Ramada hotel built there right next to the pier, so we might just get some sunshine and, wrapped up from the cold, we could walk on the prom.   Barbara and Paul agreed to spend the second day with us so I went on line and booked us a room, but not before first having a day out to Southport to look at the hotel. The day we went to view it we looked at the buffet style restaurant to see what I would be coping with. In doing so we met a lovely waitress, who on seeing why I had a need to view the place, was so reassuring. She had a lovely chat with Dave who randomly began to sing to her as she showed him where he would be having breakfast. I felt positive. We were looking forward to a holiday again although I accepted things were getting worse I just kept my expectations within my sights. Was this denial? I suppose it was but as long as we had a plan we had a future.

March 2012

So we were booked to go to Southport for two nights on March the 26th, but early on in the month things began to go pear-shaped again. I never knew what mood Dave would be in each morning and if he wouldn't, or couldn't, co-operate when I was dressing him. This was made even more difficult through lack of sleep, as his alarm would go off two or three times a night and I was exhausted. Doreen continued to come but I couldn't risk leaving her with him for long. Jeanette maintained contact and I knew she was just at the end of the phone.

On a Friday morning early that month I went to get Dave ready and was met with such pure hostility I decided to try later. He kept shouting for attention so I decided to ring Kavanagh House to ask if I could take him in early. I went up in answer to his shouting to find he was standing near the dressing table shaking with rage. The dressing table has a glass top on which stands a jug with a bowl and several framed photographs. Taking hold of the whole shelf he picked it up turned, and threw the whole thing over the bed and towards the window. The noise seemed to shock him while I stood in the doorway, fingers in my ears. He threw the whole thing away from me not towards me and I think it was pure frustration from a man who wouldn't hurt a fly.

We both sat and cried afterwards and Dave remained subdued for the rest of the morning Jeanette rang me just to see how the week had gone since her last visit and of course I had to tell her but assured her I was alright as I would be taking him in for respite shortly. She rang back a few minutes later insisting she would come to take us both to Kavanagh Place as she didn't want to risk anything happening on the journey. So we went in her car telling Dave she wanted to look around Kavanagh to see where he spent his weekends and what his room was like. He accepted that but I felt he looked so sad when we left him as though I was betraying him.

On the drive home Jeanette suddenly said to me, 'You do know it won't be long now, don't you Joan? I felt my stomach lurch.

Comments had been made about not knowing how I was coping but this was the first time a professional (whom I had come to regard as a friend to us both) had voiced what a lot of people were already thinking. I pulled myself together and casually said, 'Do you mean, before he has to go into residential care?'

She replied, 'Well I think so, don't you?'

'I suppose so', I said. Some conversations you just never forget.

That afternoon I felt dreadful, but on the Saturday I felt calmer and almost grateful that the suggestion was coming from someone else that perhaps more respite could be the answer.

Jeanette arranged a meeting between Craig (who is now assistant manager of Kavanagh place) herself, Chloe, who was nurse in charge of the Unit that day and myself. The meeting would also be attended by Jan who was an assessor from St. Helens Continuing Health Care Funding Office. We had secured funding for respite the previous year and I presumed this meeting would be regarding Dave's future as a resident at Kavanagh Place.

From the start of the meeting I sensed that everyone was in agreement that due to the unpredictability of Dave's behaviour my safety in keeping him at home was the main issue. I think I was the only one unprepared for this, even though Jeanette had been giving out warning signals. Jan was very patient, understanding my reluctance as I repeatedly asked whether I would be able to bring him home for an overnight stay and whether I would be able to visit every day and stay as long as I wanted. I was assured I could turn up at any time I wanted day or night.

Eventually I agreed, but only after asking if I could take him on that one more holiday break to Southport and if it could be after Easter as the children were coming to visit. This was agreed as long as I rang Kavanagh and got him there as soon as I sensed any trouble. Craig then gave me his mobile number saying if I had any problems at Southport, even if it was three o clock in the morning, he would come and take us to Kavanagh Place.

So Dave had a planned admission as a resident for Friday the 13th of April. Towards the end of the meeting, by which time I couldn't stem the tears, Jan asked me how long Dave and I had been married. 'Forty nine years this August', I replied breaking down again.

At which Jan's professional mask slipped and she had to turn away to hide her tears. Pulling herself together she said, 'Can we go and meet him? I've written and spoken about him so many times but have yet to meet him'. So, bringing her colleague with her, we all went along to the Unit, Strawberry Fields, where Dave was in a great mood. It was the all singing, all dancing Dave and I think Jan could see why I was reluctant to let him go. I really can't thank everyone enough for the sensitivity with which everything was handled at the meeting that day and for the reassurance given to me throughout.

The next formality was our last home visit from Dr Frances. The visit went pretty much as usual in that Dave had a chat with her and then I did, mostly about the acceptance of Dave's future in residential care. It wasn't until she was leaving that the implications of changes ahead set in. I hadn't thought of the fact that after the last ten years both she and Jeanette would no longer be part of our lives. When she shook hands with us both I felt quite emotional, though I don't think Dave realised the finality of it all. When I did lose Dave, Dr Frances wrote me a wonderful letter in which she said, 'You and David were a beacon of inspiration. I shall carry the experience of having shared a little of your joys and sadness with me for the rest of my career'.

Saying goodbye to Jeanette was so difficult too although I knew our paths would cross again through support groups etc. It was truly the end of an era but I was learning to accept it as just a different stage. Little did I know how short a stage it would be.

Southport

The couple of weeks before going to Southport were relatively quiet, but in a sad sort of way, as Dave didn't seem particularly interested in anything. The weather that March of 2012 was exceptionally warm and sunny, warm enough for Dave to be able to open the patio doors and sit outside on the swing seat listening to his music. One morning I was sitting with him on the swing when, in a very pensive mood, he took my hand

and said, 'Joan'.   There was a long pause after I answered him before he said quite clearly, 'Will we always be together?'

I couldn't believe it. What was going on in that head of his? How much did he understand? I replied, 'Yes , of course'.   But I had always been truthful with him regarding his care so I followed it up with, ' Things are becoming a little more difficult and I am getting tired these days so I may need more respite but this will always be your home, and yes we will always be together'.   I figured that when he was in Kavanagh I would be spending so much time there that, we would indeed always be together.   This answer seemed to placate him as he squeezed my hand and sat contentedly if a little seriously and continued to swing. A poignant memory for me.

On March 23rd we set off for Southport and Dave knew we were going on a little holiday but, in retrospect, I'm not sure if he understood that we were calling at Sue and Richard's on the way as they lived in Southport. Although we saw a lot of them in the early days of the Alzheimer's Southport group and had many meals together at each other's houses. In fact we had become quite a foursome; we hadn't seen one another for some time. As soon as we entered the house he became agitated and couldn't settle or sit down. He greeted Sue with a very nervous smile and not the usual hug. I didn't think it was good for Richard to see him like this. We did suggest sitting outside but he just wanted to go. Discussing this with Sue recently, I said I wondered what had triggered it. 'Alzheimer's', she said quite simply.

Having got him out of the house and into the car I drove off, planning to abort the holiday plan and go home, but when I got to the main road I turned right towards Southport and pulled up to talk when it was safe and he had calmed down. I suggested we call at the hotel and cancel the booking, but by the time we got there he was in a different frame of mind again so I took a chance and checked in. He loved the room but we went straight out as it was such a sunny day. Walking towards the pier with difficulty, as he was now having mobility problems, we could hear music and in a bar underneath there was a stage with Karaoke going on. Ideal I thought and on entering someone was calling my name. It was our daughter Jane's in laws Hilda and John. They had arranged to meet some friends for lunch. So there was Dave sitting in the sun with people he knew and loved and getting into the holiday mood.

We left them to go and meet Dave's sister Barbara and Paul as planned and spent the afternoon having a very slow walk, eating fish and chips out of the paper, and enjoying an Ice cream in the sun. Noticing signs of extreme tiredness I suggested taking Dave back to the hotel where we could have coffee in the room and he could have a sleep. Barbara and I laughed as Paul having overexerted himself eating fish and chips, climbed on the king-size bed alongside Dave where they both fell asleep after a few bouts of laughter. Day one had been a huge success after all.

The dining room at breakfast was not quite as successful, as the glorious weather had meant a sudden increase in last minute bookings and the place was crowded. There was no one on the desk so, having spotted a table on the far side of the room, I made my way across holding Dave's hand. The wavy patterned carpet made him shuffle more than usual and I was thinking, 'Just let us get sat down'. As I pushed his chair towards the glass topped table his knee gave a sudden jerk toppling the whole table over, crockery, silver and all. The noise seemed tremendous but, typically British', everyone pretended not to notice. Smiling through gritted teeth I took a bow and said to anyone who cared to listen, 'Well that was a good start wasn't it?'

Two ladies immediately came to my rescue and the ice was broken. Then the waitress spotted us and came over saying to Dave, 'You remember me don't you Dave? You sang to me'. I hoped that Dave wouldn't see this as an invitation to sing as I felt we had drawn enough attention to ourselves for one meal. She was lovely though, chatting to Dave and making us feel at home and I regret not having got around to telling the manager what an asset she was.

Day two was spent pretty much the same as the first, and at the end of it I drove home thinking, 'we could do this again'. Ever the optimist.

Chapter 25

EASTER SUNDAY

We both felt much better after our mini holiday, knowing we would be seeing the family again at Easter, which was only two weeks away. This made me feel that I could cope with anything. Of course I had also become more accepting of the fact that Dave was going to be spending more time at Kavanagh from the 13th of April .I had come to view this as longer respite. The only way I could accept this was by hanging on to the fact that I could take him home for an overnight stay once a week and maybe even do anther mini break in Southport.

Easter Sunday morning changed all of that. Jane and the girls were downstairs looking for their Easter eggs when I went in to see if Dave was awake. He was awake but I couldn't read the expression on his face. What appeared to be a confused expression quickly turned to one of anger. Deciding to forego the shower, I asked if he would let me help him freshen up with some wipes but he began to lash out at me. Jane was outside the room asking if she could come in and help so, having got his boxers on him first, I stood by to see if she could help him get dressed. It was when we got him on the landing to descend the stairs that things got really difficult. He couldn't negotiate the stairs and at the same time was gripping my arm hard, becoming angrier and at times refusing to budge one way or the other.

Paul came up and somehow got around behind us to help him from the back but, as he said to Jane later, there was a point when he thought all four of us were going to come tumbling down the stairs. Having got Dave into the dining room where Millie and Annie were I thought their distraction might work, but when I gave him Easter eggs to hand over he threw them across the room. Trying to appeal to him like I did at Christmas over Sue's children I said 'Don't spoil Easter Dave, the children have travelled a long way to see you and they love you very much'.

'Well I don't love you', he shouted back. There was anger there but there was also fear as well and he knew that I knew that. I know he did.

Jane was distressed and insisted there was no way she could go home thinking I would ever attempt to get him downstairs again, so it was decided that we should ring Kavanagh Place where the staff told us to bring him in immediately. I thought we would never get him into the car as he struggled so much with Paul, accompanied by the usual bad language. We decided to sit him in the back of the car as it had child locks on and I would sit in the front with Jane. All I can remember about that journey was a rear view of him in the mirror glaring at me. We rang from outside Kavanagh so that someone would come and meet us in case we had a struggle and although he did co-operate, on entering he began to struggle again. Some staff appeared from other units going for their lunch break and were quite shocked on seeing him like this as they had only seen the sociable side of Dave. Having got him to his room the mayhem continued and as I stood crying in the doorway the most poignant memory for me was when Jane, through her tears looked up at her lovely dad and shouted, 'Who are you and what have you done with my dad?' It was heart-breaking.

We left soon after and went to Hilda and John's for an Easter Sunday dinner and so that Millie and Annie could have their Easter egg hunt, but I couldn't get the thought out of my head. How would Dave react to me when he saw me next?

Leaving it until the Tuesday before I went to see him I can't describe how anxious I felt on entering Strawberry Fields which, I suppose, was his new home now. I was full of apprehension as I entered the lounge. To my delight he stood up to greet me with the broadest of smiles and we hugged Although he wasn't distressed he wasn't quite with it either but it was a great visit as far as I was concerned and, more importantly, when it came time for me to leave he let me go with no fuss and the reassurance that I would be back the next day.

When I used to take Dave in for weekend respite I would prepare his clothes rolled in a pack, socks , boxers, T-shirt, pants and sweater all colour co-ordinated of course and with his name on. Consequently when he became a resident the first day Emma one of his carers opened his wardrobe to be faced with all his clothes she said to the other carers, 'Oh my God, I'm going to have to choose, and Joan does like everything matching'. They must have thought I was a real control freak but, wanting their loved ones to look presentable in a care home is something most carers worry about. Fortunately at Kavanagh Place there was never a need to worry about this either for me or any of the other Carers.

Sue, one of the other wives, and I often spent an afternoon with Dave and her husband Steve listening to Dave's Liverpool football song music (even though they are Manchester United fans) but a particular memory is of the four of us watching Dave's DVD of the show Les Mis, just as though we were at home. They both seemed to enjoy the music (music which I find so emotional to listen to now).

I went in one day to find Dave, not quite with it, with no focus, a little sleepy. Barry, Trish and Mark came to visit that day and I could tell by their expressions that they could see a difference in him. I asked Jan the Unit manager if he had been given any different medication and was told that he hadn't. After our visitors had gone she came into the lounge for a chat and I could tell she was observing Dave all the time.

As the days went on Dave appeared to become more sleepy, and then one day, whilst the staff were toileting him, he had a seizure. They moved him into a quiet lounge immediately and Craig came up to see to him. Dave came out of it but when I went in to the room he was having another 'absence' and Craig asked if I had ever seen him like that before. I hadn't and as they were calling Dave's name, I don't know what made me do it, but I blew a raspberry on the back of his head. I don't know if that did it but Craig laughed and said, 'Well, I've seen some ways of bringing them around but never that one'. We got him into bed and I reassured Craig and the staff that I would rather him be cared for at Kavanagh than moved to hospital.

Chapter 26

MAY 2012

Throughout early May Dave was becoming less talkative and at times asking to go back to bed. He got angry with me one day when I was trying to wake him to stimulate him. He shouted more clearly than I had heard him speak for some time, 'I WANT TO GO TO BED'. So the staff helped me get him back into bed and I got a chair alongside his bed and held his hand while we both went to sleep. I woke up after a while but Dave was still in a deep sleep. He had been quite alert that morning as his sister Barbara fed him some Weetabix. She was due to go on a trip for a long weekend so had wanted to see him before she left. I had been with him all day and when I couldn't rouse him I decided to go home. As I was leaving I turned to look at him and he gave me one of those incredible smiles, so I went back and sat with him again but he was soon asleep again. It took me a while to remember that smile, which was so important to me, as that was the last time I saw Dave awake.

There was a social event at our club organised by the 'Making Sense group. Joan and Jane organised a buffet and the Morris dancers were going to perform, including Dave's nurse Jeanette. The mini bus from Kavanagh Place was to bring some of the residents but Dave obviously wasn't well enough to go. This was the first time he had missed anything and even with all the sleeping, I didn't appreciate what was happening. I couldn't see it was the beginning of the end.

Over the years I have read so many books about dementia, and the people who are in the carers' role, some high profile authors, some not, but the most powerful passage I have ever read that describes Dave's last few weeks is from a book called *Keeper: Living with Nancy. A Journey into Alzheimer's* by Andrea Gillies - published by Short Books 2009.

'Dementia is fast becoming the condition that's quoted by the young and healthy as the disease that is most feared. It's not curable, unlike cancer. It's not able to be tackled with drastic measures, unlike heart disease and its bypasses and transplants. It's more fundamental than that. We don't have brains, we are our brains. You can lose a leg or an arm, accept the gift of another person's heart and lungs, and still be yourself. The brain is where the self-lives. Lose the use of your brain by degrees and the self is stripped away, layer by layer. In the early stages, the middle stages, even in the early part of the late stage this may well be something you are conscious of, the lights going out one by one'.

Dave's lights were going out one by one and I couldn't see it. I had decided to have a day off on the Thursday to go for lunch with some old friends in Liverpool. I arrived at our meeting place and decided to ring Kavanagh Place only to be told by Jan that Dave wasn't well but sleeping. I asked if I should come in and she said he was alright and there was no need to come in, but just to be aware that he wasn't well. Did the penny drop? No. Not until the following morning when I went in early and she asked me to come in to the office. Sitting me down she sat opposite me and told me gently, but quite clearly, that Dave was in the last stage; his swallowing was compromised and he was aspirating fluid. His body was shutting down.

I can still feel the lurch in my stomach as I remember her words. I went straight to him and sat holding his hand. He just looked as though he was in a peaceful sleep. It was suggested that I ring Sue and Jane. They could stay with me at Kavanagh place and accommodation would be found for us. It was only when I was telling them that the enormity of it all hit me. I went home to pack a bag and Jane arrived that night and Sue the following day. We were to stay with Dave until the end.

Ten years and we still couldn't believe it. When I rang his brother Derek on the Saturday morning his response was, 'He ate a bowl of Ice cream for me yesterday'. Derek and his wife Ella came straight away. We decided not to let Barbara know as she would be home on the Monday and no one knew how long it would be .It could be three weeks or a couple of days. One thing the girls and I agreed on was that we did not want drips, artificial feeding or anything invasive. This had already been discussed with Dave in the very early stage. It's not a moral issue With Alzheimer's once the swallowing has gone there is no turning back and the rest of the organs shut down. We just wanted Dave to be pain free. It was explained that his kidneys would fail and that a procedure known as 'The Liverpool

Pathway' could be put into place, keeping him pain free but letting him die a natural death. We agreed to it. Due to recent negative media reporting regarding The Liverpool Pathway I would like to point out that everything was explained to me fully in a most caring yet professional manner.

As a family I can't begin to express our gratitude for the positive 'end of life experience' the staff gave us. That few days before Dave died had so many incidents that bordered on the hysterical as we swung between tears and laughter that I felt Dave's philosophy of 'ALWAYS LOOK ON THE BRIGHT SIDE' was remaining with us.

On the Saturday morning (19th May) Craig asked if we would we like a priest to come. Knowing how important this was to Dave I agreed and explained we had already been asked but there appeared to be some difficulty in locating one. Undaunted Craig was on a mission (appropriate choice of words) to find a priest. 'Kate from the kitchen will take me to one in her car', he said. 'Her mum and dad know a priest from their church and Kate knows where to go'.

I thought Kate sounded so funny when she told me at a later date in her lovely Liverpool accent, 'There was I chopping my mushrooms, when Craig burst in telling me that he needed a priest'. Off they went only to find no answer at the presbytery. They decided to go to another church but en-route they saw Father John coming out of the newsagents, newspaper tucked under his arm. Pulling up sharply they jumped out of the car,

Craig shouting, 'Father, we need a priest, we have a dying man'.

'Take me to him', said Father John. Craig said later it looked like a scene from the film 'Sister Act'. Within half an hour an out of breath Craig appeared in the doorway of Dave's room, Father John alongside him. By this time Dave's Brother Derek and wife Ella had arrived so, at Father John's suggestion, we held hands while he gave Dave the last rites. Father John asked us how long we had been living with Alzheimer's explaining that his late father had it. He also, on noticing Dave was having his lips and mouth moistened, suggested that like his late father (who liked a drop of Scotch) it may be an idea to moisten his lips with whisky. We thought this quite funny and said that Dave wasn't that fond of whisky. Before he left Father John looked at Dave's memory board commenting on the photographs of Dave and I, taken all over the world. 'You have been blessed with having had an amazing life', he said. And we had.

After he left Craig asked, 'What did Dave like to drink Joan?'.

'Usually just beer or lager', I said. A while later we laughed when Craig brought in a bottle of Peroni Lager to moisten Dave's lips.

When Sue arrived after her long journey we all got so emotional again. Like me she had not really accepted that this was the end and had spent the night before worrying about not being there to support Sophie who was in the middle of doing her G.S.Es. Having rung the Unit manager and realising how near the end was Sue made the decision not to tell the children, but to come straight up. She said the enormity of what was happening hit her when she said to her husband, 'My dad is dying Wayne'.

I will be eternally grateful to both my sons-in-law, Paul and Wayne, for holding the fort and looking after the children, which meant my two lovely daughters were able to be with me and their dad to the end. We were given a room with a double bed and en-suite bathroom. We tried to sleep in shifts for a couple of hours, taking our mobile phones with us, so we could come straight back if there was any change.

Barry, Trish and Mark arrived bringing cream cakes to make sure we didn't go hungry. Then my brother Michael, who had always regarded Dave as an older brother, arrived with my brother-in-law Norman. Apparently on the way in Norman had asked Mike to try and keep it together for my sake and not get to emotional but on entering the room it was Norman who broke down. It was all too much and reminded him of when my sister June was at the end of her life. On the Saturday evening the 'Liverpool Pathway' Nurses came to set up the infusion pump which was a relief, as although unconscious, Dave was showing signs of discomfort. Once again I was assured that the amount of analgaesia given would only be enough to alleviate the pain and would in no way hasten Dave's death. We don't hear a lot about these nurses, trained specifically to ease any discomfort of the dying, but I have to say what a sensitive way they had of doing a difficult task. They have my utmost admiration and gratitude.

Sunday

Sunday morning dawned and we had tried to snatch a couple of hours sleep whether it be in the allocated bedroom, in a chair or on the floor, determined we would all three be with him until the end. Lesley (senior carer) appeared with tea, coffee and sausage butties which became known as Lesley's legendary sausage butties but of course cooked for us by the kitchen staff.   Sue and Jane still talk of how when feeling really grotty in the morning Lesley's appearance, with hot food and drinks accompanied by her beaming smile, always gave us a lift. Having showered and dressed we were ready to face another day sat either side or on the bed talking to Dave , the girls telling Dave how much they loved him and reminiscing about funny incidents that happened when they were younger and what an amazing Dad he had been. We didn't question whether he would be able to hear us or not, we just needed to verbalise it, although throughout his life he must have known how much we all loved him. At lunch time, once the residents had eaten, a table was set in the dining room and, while carers sat with Dave we were provided with a hot meal. In fact during our family's stay there we never once had to send out for any nourishment as it was provided for us throughout our stay because, as they kept telling us, 'You have to keep your strength up'.

Jean from next door came bringing Ian with her this time and he became very emotional on seeing Dave. I looked at him standing over Dave and remembered how, when we first met forty seven years, they were two young men swapping gardening tips and how Dave had done the labouring for Ian when he built our dining room extension. Where had all those years gone, but how amazing that they were here to support us now.

I rang my friend Sue who said she would like to come and see Dave if she could get a carer for Richard. I was concerned as to how she would feel knowing this would happen to Richard one day but she had made her own decision and wanted to give me some support. When she arrived she saw a very different Dave. It was becoming obvious that he wasn't just sleeping.

Edward, Dave's younger brother, arrived on one of his many visits in between his shifts as a carer and, while he and I sat either side of the bed, Dave suddenly opened his eyes wide and literally lurched himself towards me where I held him briefly in my arms. He immediately relaxed again with my arm underneath his head. Edward was urging Dave to fight, seeing this as a sign, but whatever it was Dave had gone back into his world and I asked if we couldn't just let him go, telling Dave that it would be alright to let go with our love. Someone asked if I wanted to move my arm from underneath his head, but I just wanted to hold him.

Later in the afternoon our old friends Pat, Arth, Pat Parr, Marj and Jim came together, knowing they had come to say goodbye. I found this so hard and very emotional as they approached him one by one all in their different ways; stroking his head telling him what a good mate he had been, how everyone loved him and assuring him how they would look after me when he had gone. The tears flowed freely as we all hugged one another as they left.

It was a very emotional day, and then in the evening Jan, the Unit manager appeared, although she was officially off duty. She said she just wanted to see if we were alright, but stayed for quite some time, regaling us with family tales that had us in stiches laughing as we sat around Dave. If ever she gave up nursing she could get a job as a stand up comedienne. Craig also often popped in when off duty. It was so apparent that the caring didn't stop when they went off duty.

Monday

It was decided quite early in the morning to contact Dave's sister Barbara who would be travelling home from her weekend away. The plan had been that on the Monday they would do a tour of the Cotswolds before setting off for home. Unbelievably the coach party took a unanimous vote to forgo the Cotswolds trip and return home after breakfast making sure they dropped Barbara, Paul and their luggage off at Kavanagh Place first. So they arrived at Monday lunchtime and took up residence there with us. They still talk of the holistic care all of us as a family received that week.

Martin , the manager, constantly checked in on us to make sure Dave was comfortable and that we as a family had everything we needed. Staff came in to change Dave's position and freshen him up every couple of hours, talking to him all the time and playing his favourite c.ds

Sue travelled from Southport again to give support and Barry and Trish, who had been the day before, returned with their daughters Alex and Andrea and another box of cream cakes.

The doors at the top of the corridor near Dave's room had been closed to try to discourage other residents from coming to his room, but this didn't always work, and to be honest we were glad to see them as long as nothing disturbed them. Glenda one of the other residents, would wander in saying in quite a loud voice, 'Is he still asleep?' It was her birthday that day and Sue and Jane made sure they got a present for her and often went and joined her for a cup of tea. Then there was David who had Down's syndrome and had led a very active and happy life in recent years but had now developed Alzheimer's. This meant he talked less but it certainly didn't stop him singing and his favourite song was ' Happy Birthday'. Many times Sue or Jane would step out of the room feeling devastated and then they would hear the shuffling of feet and the strains of 'Happy Birthday' being sung reducing them to giggles. He also found a way of sidling into the room shushing us, finger on lips just to look at Dave. 'Ahh!' he would say and then sidle out again in case anyone saw him. One particular night, leaving Barbara and Paul sitting with Dave, I went out to comfort the girls and all three of us had broken down when along sauntered David. I think he must have thought we were laughing and he joined us with the most infectious laugh which turned our tears to laughter leaving us breathless and concerned for him, as once he started these bouts of laughter he couldn't stop. He was a star and kept us going that week, I say 'was' as sadly David died six months after my Dave.

Tuesday

Barbara and Paul had slept on a chair and couch, the girls and I taking turns with the bed though Jane preferred making a bed up on the floor. Derek and Ella came and Edward had taken leave of absence so he could be with us.I could tell the girls were missing their husbands and children and Sue was feeling guilty for not letting her children know that Granddad was dying but was wanting to protect them at exam time. Paul had tried to prepare Millie and Annie. They were in constant contact but the strain was beginning to show.

Throughout the day the staff came in to see us often, including Paul the physiotherapist and Kaylee a senior carer. The majority of the staff were very young and some had never experienced death before, so it was hard for them too especially as they had grown so close to Dave and regarded him as a real character. That morning when they first came in one of the carers

Paul visibly cringed when he said to Jane, 'Sorry for your loss'.

'Its ok', she said smiling and he knew that we knew exactly what he meant.

Sue, (I know so many Sues), who, of course, was there so much as Steve was a resident, was constantly in and out seeing if we needed anything and little did we know that Steve would follow Dave three months later. When I heard about this I was reminded of the words of Sue, Richard's wife, when she had said, 'There is no escape from this disease. No miraculous cures, no good endings, life cannot be resumed. It picks them off one by one like sitting ducks in a fairground game. Always hitting the target, never missing.'

Donna was on nights that night, another carer whom Dave had a great rapport with. A decision was being made as to whether it would disturb Dave to change his clothes. I could tell she thought he would feel better so, at her suggestion, his t-shirt was cut up the back when being taken off to cause the minimum discomfort. He always looked more comfortable when freshened up.

That night, or early in the morning, Jane came back into the room to find me alone with Dave holding his hands and talking to him. She suggested I had some time alone with him and I agreed because I realised I had never been alone with him the last few days. So I talked to him about what a great marriage we'd had with its ups and downs, like everyone had. How blessed we had been with our children and grandchildren and how lucky we had been to have seen so much of the world in our travels. Most of all I told him how amazing he had been throughout his struggle and his fight against this dreadful disease (all the bad bits forgotten). For a quiet man, there would be people we had met from all over the world who would remember him and his courage. I was glad I had that quiet time with him.

Wednesday 23rd May

Another exhausting day dawned. Paul and Barbara had stayed another night but decided to go home for a shower and change of clothes. We had our usual sausage butties from Lesley and put Dave's music on.

Martin paid his usual morning visit, as did Craig.

Jane sat on the bed and began to massage Dave's hands and arms (he must have smelt beautiful that day) while Sue sat on the other side, both of them talking to him and each other. The day seemed much like previous days other than his change in colour. Lunch time came around and Kate wheeled in a trolley with hot pot and drinks etc. Dave's breathing began to be more laboured so Craig was sent for while Dave's observations were taken. 'It's going to be soon', said Craig. 'Just hold his hands'.

'Love you Dad', was all I could hear from the girls and at ten past one it was over. As described in the book 'The Keeper' his light had finally gone out. My lovely Dave had gone. His battle was finished and just the three of us were with him.

EPILOGUE

Craig and staff entered the room to prepare him for being taken from Kavanagh place, having given us some time to sit for a while with Dave. There were tears and hugs as we thanked them for everything they had done. The words of thanks seemed so inadequate. As we left the room Sue and Jane urged them to play Dave's Liverpool songs. We sat in one of the lounges and as often happens at times like this the room was entered by someone who hadn't heard the news. Moving the occasional furniture out of the room, Jay, one of the activity, staff smiled at us and said 'Happy Times'. Happy times was what they called Wednesday afternoons when a team of volunteers came in for musical therapy and Jay was preparing the room.

'You haven't heard have you Jay?' said Sue. I can still see the smile disappear from his face and the crestfallen look as he tried to apologise. Reassuring him with a hug we saw the funny side of the way he entered the room. Jay was another one of Dave's favourite people who worked alongside Paul the physiotherapist. When we returned to his room Dave was lying peacefully, with the colourful blanket made of family photo's for his 70th birthday spread over him.

His music was playing and even though the curtains were drawn the sunlight streamed in.

His funeral at our parish church St Mary's Birchley was amazing. He entered the church to his favourite hymn, 'How Great Thou Art', to be received by my cousin

Father Tony, who was given permission to do this by Father Bernard our Parish priest. He was carried in by his brother Edward, my cousin Barry, friends Arth and Jim and Dave's nephews Andrew and Stephen. Our brother-in-law Paul was the Eucharistic minister and he read the following Eulogy which he had written.

DAVID CRANK 1941-2012

'Today we come together to say a physical farewell to David Crank. We come in a spirit of hope, a spirit of love, a spirit of faith and a spirit of thankfulness. Because Dave is out of sight he will never be out of our minds and hearts. I am proud to speak to you today.
Dave was a happy man, born in Liverpool on 28th August 1941, he had two brothers Derek and Edward and one sister Barbara. His early education was at St John The Evangelist Kirkdale, at which church he was an altar boy. From there, after passing the 11 plus, he went to Evered Avenue Technical college. After his apprenticeship he pursued a career in engineering.

Dave was a keen Liverpool Football Club supporter. By now I am quite sure he has had quite a word in you know whose ear (well they do need all the help they can get).

I am very lucky to have Barbara my wife because she survived David pushing her down the street in her pram, as David would jump into the pram with her, and down the street he would go. She also said that David was tight with pocket money when he began work. (She did forgive him).

Dave met Joan the love of his life, when he was working in Blue Cap foods. He went into the shop were Joan worked every day, but it took him two years to ask her out, on her last day in the shop at her leaving do. He must have thought it's now or never.

They married on 31st August 1963 at Our Lady of The Assumption Church Gatacre Liverpool, first living in Wavertree and then moving to Billinge in 1965. They were in the same house for 46 years next door to Aunty Jean and Uncle Ian.

Joan, my next words are directed to you personally. Dave Crank was besotted with you and loved you from the first time he set eyes on you, and that love grew and grew more deeply and intensely as the years moved on, but I'm sure you knew that.

They had two daughters Susan (Sunday name) and Jane, both of whom he loved so deeply and was so proud of. To you, your mum wants to say, she could not have done what she did for your Dad without the sure knowledge of your love and support.

Dave's family was everything to him. He was a proud and happy man. Never happier than when he was with you. There have been many happy moments recalled over the last few days since David died. Once when Dave drank some Paracetamol mixture for Jane so she could be discharged from hospital quicker. Putting up the school netball post so that Sue and her friends could get plenty of practice.'

Paul went on to say what a much respected father-in-law Dave was to Wayne and Paul and how he loved his grandchildren more than they would ever know urging them to keep him in their hearts.

Speaking of what an important part Billinge and the parish of St Mary's had played in Dave's life, Paul mentioned how our friends had become like extended family and what a major part Dave had played in village life. Being Father Christmas, involved with youth, the social club and working for Riding for the Disabled. He talked of our holidays and the funny incidents around them and he mentioned how much support we had from the various groups we had been involved with.

Finishing by thanking Dr Linden and carers, he said of Kavanagh Place 'The last few months of David's life were made so much easier for him and his family by the kind care, attention and love given without reservations from all at Kavanagh Place. Words cannot express our thanks for all you did for Dave, even to the extent of kidnapping the local priest in the street to bless Dave and the family. The staff of Kavanagh Place are a living example of the gospel message, 'To love one another as I have loved you'.

Dave you will be missed more than you will ever know and the world will be a sorrier place without you. Thank you Lord for giving Dave to us. So, in the spirit of faith, the spirit of hope , the spirit of love and the spirit of thankfulness we now give him back to you, where he will rest in peace forever.'

The church was so crowded that people were standing in the aisles and up in the choir as well as the porch. The Mass was so personal with family and friends involvement, Jean and Ian doing the Offertory procession.

Whilst sitting outside in the car, we were amazed when our retired priest, Father Ashton came to speak to us. At ninety plus years, he had travelled from Cheshire to attend the Requiem Mass. As he held hands with Sue, Jane and myself, he paid tribute to what a good man Dave had been.

A man of humility, Dave would have been astounded.

After a short service at the Crematorium conducted by Father Tony who commented on how, once again, a full house with standing room only proved how loved and respected Dave was. He entered the crematorium to music from his favourite DVD Les'Mis 'I dreamed a dream', but when he left it was to his old favourite, often sung either when happy or when things got difficult. Yes it was 'Always Look On The Bright Side Of Life'. I can still see the look on Dave's niece Sara's face when I turned around as the music started up. A mixture of surprise and pleasure. He left people smiling to the end.

We returned to St Mary's Social Club where there must have been 200 people waiting for us, all by invitation on the back of the order of service. Jennifer, the caterer, did an incredible feat of creating a sort of rolling buffet as we had no real idea how many would come back. Dave stories were swapped. The grandchildren took around 'memories of granddad' books for people to write in, which I will treasure for the rest of my life.

We received two hundred and eighty mass and sympathy cards and to Alzheimer's Research, donations amounting to two thousand pounds.

So what of me now? I have to keep busy or I would fall apart, I miss him so much. Then there are the days when I'm enjoying coffee, toast and a bit of morning telly feeling relaxed and then the guilt comes; because I can only do this as I haven't got the responsibility for caring for Dave any more.

I am still involved with support groups. I am a Trustee with the St. Helens' 'Mind' charity, involved with Joan and Jane's 'Making Sense' group, now part of the Hargreaves Dementia Trust, and still calling into see Joanne and the ladies at the Carers Centre. I am now a voluntary worker for the Alzheimer's Society, helping Denise run the Thursday morning group and soon starting up a new group for younger people with dementia. Having recently been invited onto a panel involved with improving strategies for speeding up diagnosis and maintaining good quality care in the Five Boroughs Partnership NHS Trust; it's good to know there is an aim to improve standards even more .

This is not because I'm clinging on to the past. I do feel that I can empathise with other carers but mostly it is because I love trying to connect or converse with people who have this awful condition. If I see a spark in their eyes or a smile from someone who has stopped communicating it makes my day. I'm no expert but ten years of living with it must count for something surely. I have made so many new friends, as well as keeping my old friends, that my support is wonderful as I'm still hearing from people worldwide who we met on our travels.

Ironically I finished writing this book, which started out as a bit of a diary, this week, the week of my seventieth birthday. Sue and Jane travelled with the grandchildren through the snow and ice to give me a wonderful family party and it's been a week of celebrating with different groups. So much for not wanting a big party.

A new beginning perhaps. I start a creative writing course that Sue is facilitating at Southport tomorrow, but I don't' think I will become a writer of steamy novels. I want to be brave enough to try a cruise alone on a good old Fred Olsen ship from Liverpool, as Dave and I met so many interesting people who do travel alone. I have just had a holiday over Christmas with Barry, Trish and family which got my first Christmas over and was so relaxing.

It's been an incredible journey. I hate that expression, but I knew I'd use it in the end. It has been a journey that has enriched my life.

A couple of years ago Sue, Richard, Dave and I were wandering around a garden centre when we bumped into a lady whom we hadn't seen for quite some time. She had been bereaved the previous year, her husband having had dementia. Both Dave and Richard had become worse since we last met her and, in fact, Richard wandered off as we were talking. I think there was a bit of eye rolling from Sue when the lady said, 'Oh, don't Sue. It is so awful when they have gone. I would have him back tomorrow if I could'. This left us both feeling uncomfortable.

'Don't feel guilty Sue', I said as we left. Every person with this illness is so different and both our partners were demanding, but that didn't mean we loved them any the less. Would I wish Dave back into this world, much as I miss him, to suffer as he did? The answer is an emphatic no. God knows how much torment he was going through with whatever was going on in his brain.

Dave is at peace now after a determined battle to live as normal a life as possible. We had a wonderful life and wonderful family and friends and, although I have my dark days, I know he has left a legacy of love and hope and, those two words, spoken of at the beginning 'Acceptance and Gratitude.'

Goodnight Dave, the love of my life. Sleep easy.